Cardiac Arrhythmias

# Cardiac Arrhythmias

*Practical Notes on
Interpretation and Treatment*

**David H. Bennett** MD, MRCP

*Consultant Cardiologist,
Regional Cardiac Centre, Wythenshawe Hospital,
Manchester*

Second Edition

**WRIGHT**

Bristol
1985

*Published by*
John Wright & Sons Ltd, Techno House, Redcliffe Way, Bristol BS1 6NX, England


*First edition*, 1981
*Second edition,* 1985


*British Library Cataloguing in Publication Data*

Bennett, David H.
    Cardiac arrhythmias: practical notes on
    interpretation and treatment. − 2nd ed.
    1. Arrhythmia
    I. Title
    616.1′28   RC685.A65


ISBN 0 7236 0845 8

*Printed in Great Britain by*
John Wright & Sons (Printing) Ltd, at the Stonebridge Press, Bristol BS4 5NU

# Preface to the Second Edition

The purpose of this second edition remains the same: to provide a practical guide to the diagnosis, investigation and management of the main cardiac arrhythmias with particular emphasis on the problems commonly encountered in practice.

The author is grateful for the generous reviews of the first edition and has made a point of responding to suggestions reviewers have made. Since the first edition, new anti-arrhythmic drugs have been introduced, a substantial amount of new information about the older drugs has been acquired, approaches to the management of ventricular arrhythmias (particularly in acute infarction) have been modified and there have been important improvements in cardiac pacing.

Accordingly, the sections relating to treatment have been extensively updated and expanded. Elsewhere, changes to the text have been made to highlight areas where there are common pitfalls.

A summary has been added at the end of each chapter to draw attention to the main points and to highlight those facts of practical importance that are often forgotten or neglected.

A number of new ECGs and illustrations have been added and the quiz section at the end of the book has been increased in size.

D.H.B.

# Preface to the First Edition

The purpose of this book is to describe the main cardiac arrhythmias, with particular emphasis on the problems commonly encountered in their interpretation, and to discuss the practical aspects of current methods of investigation and treatment. Information of purely academic value has not been included.

This book is intended to fill the gap between those textbooks that cover only the basics of arrhythmias and those that are written for the cardiac electrophysiologist. It has been written with junior hospital doctors in mind. They receive little formal training in the management of cardiac arrhythmias and yet, because prompt action is often required, the onus of diagnosis and treatment usually falls on them. It should also be of interest to medical students, who themselves will soon be responsible for dealing with arrhythmias, to nurses working in coronary and intensive care units and to physicians who want a brief review of the practical aspects of cardiac arrhythmias.

I would like to thank the cardiac technicians, coronary care nurses and medical staff at Wythenshawe Hospital for their help. I am particularly grateful to my colleagues, Dr Colin Bray and Dr Christopher Ward.

Thanks are also due to Mrs Mary Rooney for typing the manuscript and to the Wythenshawe Hospital Medical Illustration Department.

Finally, I would like to acknowledge the distractions provided by my family, Irene, Samantha and Sally, to whom this book is dedicated.

D.H.B.

# Contents

| | | |
|---|---|---|
| 1 | Sinus Rhythm | 1 |
| 2 | Ectopic Beats | 4 |
| 3 | Escape Beats | 15 |
| 4 | Bundle Branch Blocks | 18 |
| 5 | Ventricular Tachycardia | 24 |
| 6 | Tachycardias of Supraventricular Origin | 34 |
| 7 | Pre-excitation Syndromes | 56 |
| 8 | Tachycardias with Broad Ventricular Complexes | 65 |
| 9 | Atrioventricular Block | 72 |
| 10 | Sick Sinus Syndrome | 83 |
| 11 | Arrhythmias in Myocardial Infarction | 90 |
| 12 | Anti-arrhythmic Drugs | 105 |
| 13 | Cardioversion | 115 |
| 14 | Cardiac Arrest | 119 |
| 15 | Temporary Cardiac Pacing | 124 |
| 16 | Long Term Cardiac Pacing | 132 |
| 17 | Digoxin Toxicity | 150 |
| 18 | Ambulatory ECG Monitoring | 154 |
| 19 | Intracardiac Electrophysiological Testing | 157 |
| 20 | Arrhythmias for Interpretation: a Quiz | 168 |
| | Index | 193 |

# Note

Unless otherwise indicated, the electrocardiograms in this book have been recorded at a paper speed of 25 mm/s. At this speed, each large square represents 0·2 s and each small square represents 0·04 s.

Heart rate (beats/minute) can be calculated by dividing the number of large squares between two consecutive complexes into 300, or by dividing the number of small squares between two complexes into 1500.

In order to include all the necessary features in the electrocardiograms, some records have had to be reduced in size.

*Chapter* **1**

# Sinus Rhythm

The sinus node is the primary pacemaker of the heart, initiating the electrical activity that leads to the orderly activation of atrial and then ventricular myocardium during each heart beat. Sinus node activity does not register on the electrocardiogram (ECG).

Atrial activity, the P wave, can be seen in most ECG leads (*Fig.* 1.1). Sometimes the P wave is of low amplitude and it may be necessary to inspect all leads of the ECG to establish that the patient is in sinus rhythm (*Fig.* 1.2).

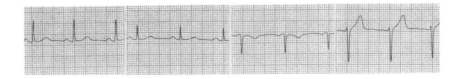

*Fig.* 1.1. Sinus rhythm (leads I, AVF, AVR and V2). Atrial activity is clearly seen in the limb leads but is only just discernible in V2.

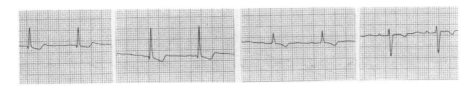

*Fig.* 1.2. Sinus rhythm with low amplitude P waves (leads I, II, III and V1). Atrial activity is only clearly seen in V1.

Atrial activation spreads from the sinus node, which lies at the junction of the superior vena cava and right atrium, in an inferior direction. The P wave, therefore, is upright in leads II, III and AVF, which are orientated towards the inferior surface of the heart, and is inverted in AVR, which is orientated towards the superior heart surface (*Fig.* 1.1). If the P wave does not have these characteristics then, even though each ventricular complex is preceded by a P wave, the rhythm is abnormal (*Fig.* 1.3).

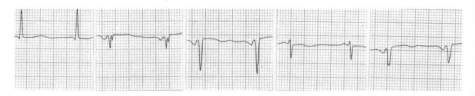

*Fig.* 1.3. Junctional rhythm (leads I, II, III, AVR, AVF): a P wave precedes each QRS complex but is superiorly directed.

The atrioventricular (AV) node delays the transmission of the activating impulse from atria to ventricles. This is reflected by the PR interval, which is measured from the onset of the P wave to the onset of the ventricular complex. The normal PR interval ranges from 0·12 to 0·21 s. It shortens with increasing heart rate.

After traversing the AV node, the electrical impulse is conducted very rapidly by the bundle of His and right and left bundle branches to the ventricular myocardium. Ventricular activation is represented by the QRS complex which, in the absence of bundle branch block, should be less than 0·08 s in duration.

## SINUS BRADYCARDIA

This is defined as sinus rhythm at a rate less then 60/min (*Fig.* 1.4). It may be physiological, as in athletes, or secondary to acute myocardial infarction, sick sinus syndrome or beta-adrenoceptor blocking drugs. Noncardiac disorders such as myxoedema, jaundice and raised intracranial pressure can also cause sinus bradycardia.

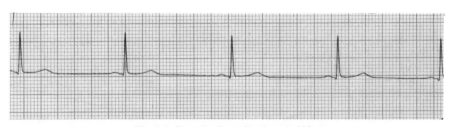

*Fig.* 1.4. Sinus bradycardia. Rate is 48/min.

## SINUS TACHYCARDIA

This is defined as sinus rhythm at a rate greater than 100/min (*Fig.* 1.5). Sinus tachycardia is caused by exercise, anxiety or any disorder that increases sympathetic nervous system activity. Occasionally it may be due to a primary disorder of the sinus node (sinus node re-entry).

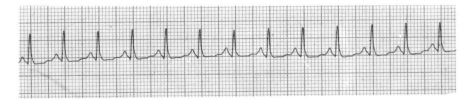

*Fig.* 1.5. Sinus tachycardia during exercise (lead II). The rate is 150/min.

At rest the sinus node rate is seldom above 120/min unless the patient is very ill. In contrast, atrial flutter with 2 : 1 AV block often leads to a heart rate of 140–160/min and can easily be mistaken for sinus tachycardia (*see* Chapter 6).

## SINUS ARRHYTHMIA

Normally there are only minor changes in rate during sinus rhythm. In sinus arrhythmia there are alternating periods of slowing and increasing sinus node rate. Usually the rate increases during inspiration (*Fig.* 1.6). Sinus arrhythmia is most commonly seen in the young.

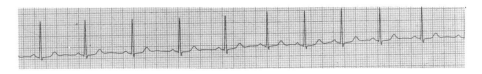

*Fig.* 1.6. Sinus arrhythmia.

## Main Points

1. For sinus rhythm, an inferiorly directed P wave (i.e. upright in leads III and AVF) must precede each QRS complex.

2. If AV conduction is normal, the duration of the PR interval will be between 0·12 and 0·21 s.

3. Normal intraventricular conduction results in a QRS complex whose duration will be less than 0·08 s.

4. In cases of apparent sinus tachycardia at rest, atrial flutter should be excluded.

# Chapter 2

# Ectopic Beats

Ectopic beats may arise from the atria, AV junction (i.e. AV node plus bundle of His) or ventricles (*Figs.* 2.1, 2.2, 2.3). For practical purposes, the terms ectopic beat, extrasystole and premature contraction are interchangeable.

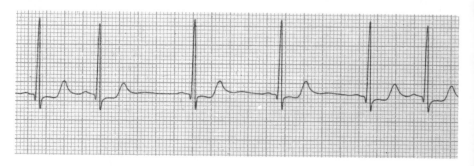

*Fig.* 2.1. Atrial ectopic beats (second and sixth beats). The ectopic P waves differ slightly in shape from those of sinus origin.

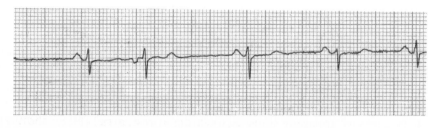

*Fig.* 2.2. The second beat is a junctional ectopic beat (lead III). The junctional focus has activated the atria as well as the ventricles, resulting in an inverted P wave which precedes the QRS complex.

Ectopic beats are premature. Thus, the interval between the ectopic beat and the preceding beat (i.e. the coupling interval) is always shorter than the cycle length of the dominant rhythm. This fact is often forgotten, with the result that other beats with abnormal configurations, i.e. escape beats (*see* Chapter 3) and intermittent bundle branch block (*see* Chapter 4)

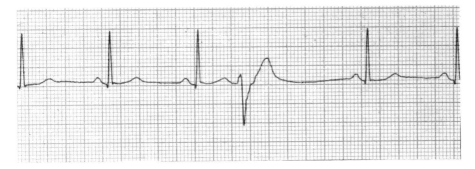

*Fig.* 2.3. The fourth beat is a ventricular ectopic beat.

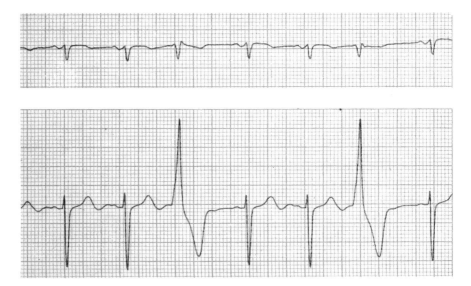

*Fig.* 2.4. Simultaneous recording of leads V1 and V2. The third and sixth beats are unifocal ventricular ectopic beats. Their ventricular origin is not apparent in lead V1 but is obvious in V2.

are misinterpreted as ectopic beats. Whereas suppression of ectopic beats may be desirable, attempts to suppress escape beats and beats with bundle branch block can be dangerous.

Usually, ectopic beats arising from the same focus have the same coupling interval and configuration (*Fig.* 2.4).

The site of origin of an ectopic beat can be ascertained from careful examination of the ECG. It cannot be stressed too strongly that a single rhythm strip does not always reveal the diagnostic clues and that scrutiny of simultaneous recordings of several ECG leads is often necessary (*Figs.* 2.4 and 2.5).

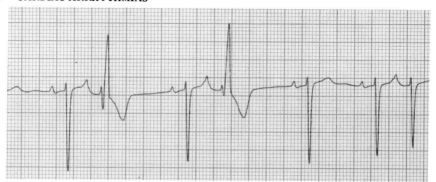

*Fig.* 2.5.   Atrial ectopic beats are superimposed on the T waves of the first, third and sixth ventricular complexes (lead V1). It can be seen how the T waves of these beats are modified by comparing them with the T wave of the fifth ventricular complex which is not followed by an atrial
ectopic. The first two atrial ectopic beats are aberrantly conducted, resulting in right bundle
branch block.

## ATRIAL ECTOPIC BEATS

These are recognized by a P wave which is premature and, because the
source and hence direction of atrial activation differ from that during
sinus rhythm, these P waves will often be of abnormal shape (*Fig.* 2.1).
Ectopic P waves may be smaller than normal, and because they are premature they may be superimposed on the T wave of the preceding beat.
Careful examination of the ECG is essential to detect ectopic P waves;
frequently they are best shown in lead V1 (*Figs.* 2.5, 2.6).

Usually an atrial ectopic beat will be conducted to the ventricles in the
same manner as if the atria had been activated by the sinus node. Thus,
the PR interval and QRS complex of the ectopic beat will be identical to
those during sinus rhythm (*Fig.* 2.1). If the QRS complex during sinus
rhythm shows bundle branch block, then so will the QRS complex in the
ectopic beat.

Sometimes, however, atrial ectopic beats, especially those that arise
very early in the cardiac cycle, may encounter either an AV junction or
bundle branch which has not yet recovered from conduction of the last
atrial impulse and is, therefore, partially or completely refractory to
excitation. Partial and complete refractoriness of the AV junction will
result in prolongation of the PR interval and blocked atrial ectopic beats,
respectively (*Figs.* 2.6–2.8). Blocked atrial ectopics have on occasion been
erroneously taken as an indication for cardiac pacing! Partial or complete
refractoriness of one or other bundle branch (it is usually the right bundle)
will lead to correspondingly partial or complete bundle branch block
(*Fig.* 2.7). This phenomenon of functional bundle branch block is referred
to as 'phasic aberrant intraventricular conduction'. The practical significance of this phenomenon is that the resultant QRS complexes are broad
and can therefore mimic ventricular ectopic beats.

Atrial ectopic beats are often benign. If they are frequent, however,
they may clinically mimic atrial fibrillation, and may herald its onset. When

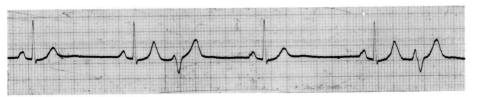

*Fig.* 2.6. The third and sixth beats are atrial ectopic beats. The premature P waves are super-imposed on the preceding T wave, as can be seen by comparing the T waves of sinus beats preceding and not preceding ectopic beats. The ectopic beats show first degree AV block and phasic aberrant conduction.

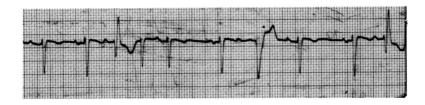

*Fig.* 2.7. Frequent atrial ectopic beats (lead V1). The seventh beat is an atrial ectopic beat conducted with left bundle branch block and marked prolongation of the PR interval. The third and tenth beats are atrial ectopic beats conducted with right bundle branch block and slight prolongation of the PR interval.

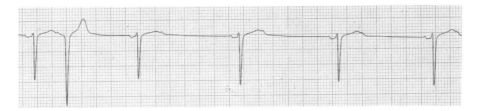

*Fig.* 2.8. Atrial ectopic beats are superimposed on the T wave of each ventricular complex. The first atrial ectopic is conducted with partial left bundle branch block. The other atrial ectopic beats are not conducted to the ventricles.

frequent atrial ectopic beats occur in patients with heart disease, especially valve disorders, myocardial infarction, cardiomyopathy or following cardiac surgery, treatment with digoxin should be considered so that the ventricular rate will be controlled should atrial fibrillation occur.

## AV JUNCTIONAL ECTOPIC BEATS

AV junctional beats used to be referred to as 'nodal' beats. It is now appreciated that at least part of the AV node is not capable of pacemaker activity and that it is not possible to distinguish between beats of AV nodal and His bundle origin. Hence the more general term 'AV junction'.

AV junctional ectopic beats are recognized by a premature QRS complex similar to that occurring in sinus rhythm. The atria as well as the ventricles may be activated by the junctional focus, leading to an inverted P wave (i.e. negative in leads II, III and AVF) which may precede, follow or be buried within the QRS complex, depending on the relative speeds of conduction from AV junction to ventricles and from AV junction to atria (*Fig.* 2.2).

AV junctional ectopic beats are not as common as atrial or ventricular ectopics. Treatment is rarely required.

## VENTRICULAR ECTOPIC BEATS

These are recognized by a premature ventricular complex which is broad (usually $>0.12$ s), bizarre in shape and, in contrast to atrial ectopic beats, will clearly not be preceded by an ectopic P wave (*Figs.* 2.3, 2.4). The abnormal shape and prolonged duration of the ventricular complex reflect the abnormal course and consequent slowing of ventricular activation.

There are a number of different terms – important because they are of either therapeutic or diagnostic significance – used to describe ventricular ectopic beats.

### Unifocal or Multifocal

Ectopic beats with the same shape and coupling interval are assumed to arise from the same focus, whereas differing contours and coupling intervals imply more than one focus (*Figs.* 2.4, 2.9).

### Early Ventricular Ectopic Beats

Ectopic beats which occur very early in the cardiac cycle will be super-imposed on the T wave of the preceding beat and are described as 'R on T' (*Fig.* 2.10). Most episodes of ventricular fibrillation and many episodes of ventricular tachycardia are initiated by 'R on T' ectopics (though by no means do all 'R on T' ectopic beats precipitate these arrhythmias).

### Late Ventricular Ectopic Beats

A ventricular ectopic beat which occurs late in the cardiac cycle may fall, by chance, immediately after a P wave initiated by sinus node activity (the P wave will therefore be normal in timing and configuration). This is referred to as an 'end-diastolic' ventricular ectopic beat (*Fig.* 2.11). This situation, in which the atrial impulse will clearly not be conducted to the ventricles, must not be confused with an ectopic atrial beat with aberrant conduction, in which case, of course, the P wave will be premature.

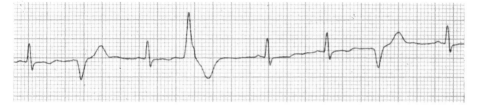

*Fig.* 2.9. Multifocal ventricular ectopic beats. The second ventricular ectopic beat has a different shape and coupling interval from the first and third ectopic beats.

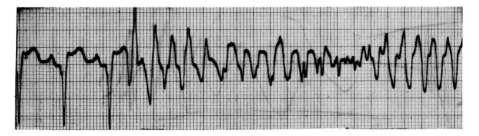

*Fig.* 2.10. An 'R on T' ventricular ectopic beat initiates ventricular fibrillation.

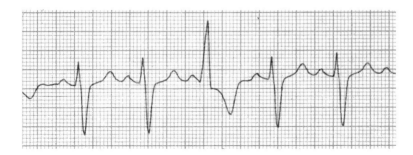

*Fig.* 2.11 The third beat is an end-diastolic ventricular ectopic beat. It is preceded by a *normally* timed P wave.

Because the initial upstroke of a ventricular ectopic beat may be slurred like a delta wave (*see* Chapter 7), end-diastolic ventricular ectopic beats can mimic the Wolff–Parkinson–White syndrome (*Fig.* 2.12).

### Interpolated Ventricular Ectopic Beats

Usually there is a pause after a ventricular ectopic beat before the next beat. When there is no such pause and the ectopic beat is thus sandwiched between two normal beats, the ectopic beat is said to be 'interpolated' (*Fig.* 2.13).

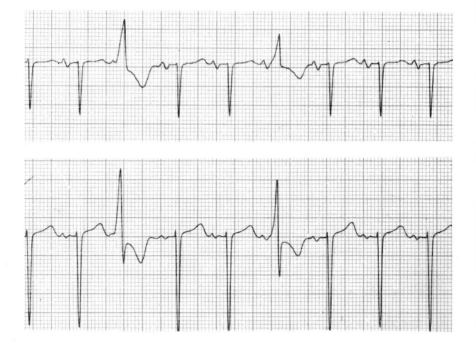

*Fig.* 2.12. Simultaneous recording of leads V1 and V2. Two end-diastolic ventricular ectopic beats. The second, mimicking the Wolff–Parkinson–White syndrome.

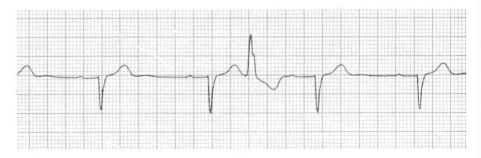

*Fig.* 2.13. Interpolated ventricular beat. The subsequent PR interval is prolonged due to retrograde concealed conduction.

## Frequency

Ventricular ectopic beats are usually quantified in terms of the number occurring per minute.

When an ectopic beat follows each sinus beat the term bigeminy is applied (*Fig.* 2.14). If an ectopic follows a pair of normal beats, there is trigeminy. When two ectopics occur in succession (*Fig.* 2.15) they are referred to as a couplet, and when there are more than two ectopic beats in succession the group is termed a salvo or ventricular tachycardia (*see* Chapter 5).

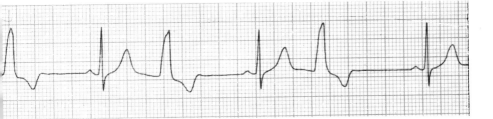

*Fig.* 2.14. Ventricular bigeminy.

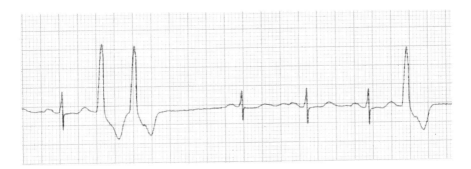

*Fig.* 2.15. The first sinus beat is followed by a couplet of ventricular ectopic beats.

## Atrial Activity

The pattern of atrial activity following a ventricular ectopic beat depends on whether or not the AV junction transmits the ventricular impulse back to the atria. If this occurs, the result is an inverted P wave which is often superimposed on and may be concealed by the ventricular ectopic beat (*Fig.* 2.16).

When the AV junction does not transmit the ventricular impulse to the atria, atrial activity proceeds independently of ventricular activity; it is only in these cases that a ventricular impulse will be followed by a full compensatory pause (*Figs.* 2.3, 2.4).

Sometimes a ventricular impulse only partially penetrates the AV junction. Particularly with interpolated ventricular ectopics, the subsequent atrial impulse arising from sinus node activation may find the AV junction partially refractory and be conducted with a prolonged PR interval (*Fig.* 2.13). The significance of this phenomenon of 'retrograde concealed conduction' is that the prolonged PR interval in these circumstances does not indicate AV node disease, and if the phenomenon is observed in the first beat after a tachycardia, a ventricular origin for the tachycardia can be inferred (*see* Chapter 8).

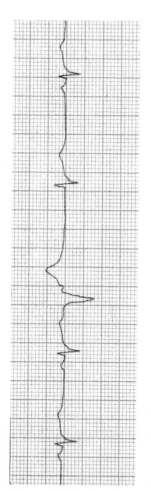

Fig. 2.16. The third beat is a ventricular ectopic beat which has been conducted back to the atria, resulting in an inverted P wave (lead AVF). The ectopic beat is followed by a junctional escape beat.

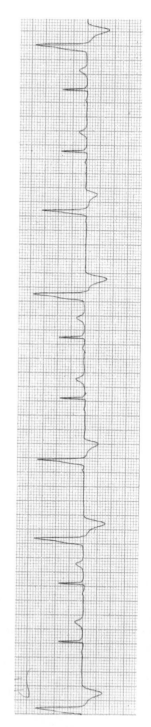

Fig. 2.17. Ventricular parasystole. The ectopic beats have a variable coupling interval. The intervals between ectopic beats are multiples of 1·18 s. The fifth and ninth beats are fusion beats.

## Parasystole

As stated above, unifocal ventricular ectopic beats have a constant coupling interval. Ventricular parasystole, a rare phenomenon, is an exception to this rule. In this arrhythmia a ventricular ectopic focus discharges regularly, undisturbed by the dominant rhythm, and will capture the ventricles provided that the ectopic discharge does not occur when the ventricles have just been activated by the dominant rhythm and are therefore refractory.

Thus, ventricular parasystole (*Fig.* 2.17) is characterized by a variable coupling interval, inter-ectopic intervals which are multiples of a common factor and, because the ventricles may by chance be simultaneously activated by both ectopic and normal pacemakers, fusion beats (complexes which in appearance are a fusion between normal and ectopic beats).

## Causes of Ventricular Ectopic Beats

Causes include acute myocardial ischaemia and infarction, chronic ischaemic heart disease, myocarditis, cardiomyopathies, mitral valve prolapse, valvular heart disease and digoxin toxicity. In some patients no cause is found.

In patients without clinically obvious heart disease, exercise ECG testing, echocardiography and ambulatory electrocardiography should be considered in the further assessment of the patient.

## Significance of Ventricular Ectopic Beats

Occasional ventricular ectopic beats at rest and even frequent unifocal ectopic beats on exercise occur in otherwise normal individuals and are not necessarily pathological or of prognostic significance.

In contrast, 'complex' ventricular ectopic beats, i.e. frequent, multifocal, 'R on T' or those that occur in salvoes are rarely found in the absence of cardiac disease and are associated with an increased cardiovascular mortality. In the setting of chronic ischaemic heart disease, a correlation between severity of left ventricular damage and frequency of ectopic beats has been demonstrated. Recent evidence, however, points to the presence of ectopic beats being an additional and independent risk factor. At present, there is no hard evidence to show that suppression or reduction in frequency of ectopic beats by anti-arrhythmic therapy improves prognosis.

Whereas ectopic beats in many individuals are asymptomatic, they may cause distressing symptoms in others, including those without evidence of structural heart disease. Symptomatic patients may be distressed by the irregularity caused by premature beats, the compensatory pause and/or 'thump' caused by increased myocardial contractility associated with the post-ectopic beat. In this minority of patients anti-arrhythmic therapy may be indicated for purely symptomatic purposes.

The significance of ventricular ectopic beats in acute myocardial infarction is discussed in Chapter 11.

# Main Points

1. Ectopic beats are premature and therefore have a coupling interval which is shorter than the cycle length of the dominant rhythm.

2. The P waves of atrial ectopic beats are often superimposed on the preceeding T wave and can easily be missed. They are usually best seen in lead V1.

3. Atrial ectopic beats may cause partial or complete AV or bundle branch block.

4. Ventricular ectopic beats cause premature, broad and bizarrely shaped QRS complexes. They are only followed by a full compensatory pause if they are not conducted to the atria.

5. Chronic ventricular ectopic beats which are frequent, multifocal, 'R on T' or occur in salvoes are associated with an increased cardiovascular mortality but there is little evidence to show that their suppression improves prognosis.

## Chapter 3

# Escape Beats

Escape beats arise from subsidiary pacemakers when the dominant pace-maker fails to discharge. In contrast to ectopic beats, they are always late, i.e. the coupling interval is greater than the cycle length of the dominant rhythm (*Figs.* 3.1, 3.3). Distinction between escape and ectopic beats is important because the former should clearly not be suppressed by drugs.

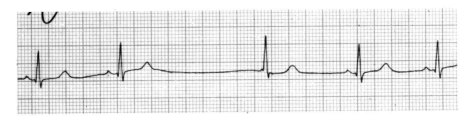

*Fig.* 3.1. The third ventricular complex is a junctional escape beat. By chance, it is superimposed on a P wave which occurs too late to capture the ventricles.

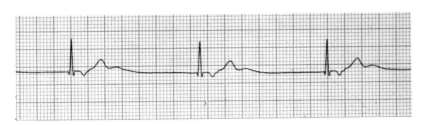

*Fig.* 3.2. Junctional escape rhythm (lead II). The junctional focus has activated the atria as indicated by the inverted P wave following each QRS complex.

Escape beats are usually of junctional origin (*Figs.* 3.1, 3.2, 3.3). Less commonly, they arise from the ventricles. The ventricular complexes of junctional escape beats are similar to those during normal rhythm. Ventricular escape beats have a similar configuration to ventricular ectopic beats (*Fig.* 3.4).

Escape beats themselves require no treatment. If treatment is indicated, it is to accelerate the basic rhythm.

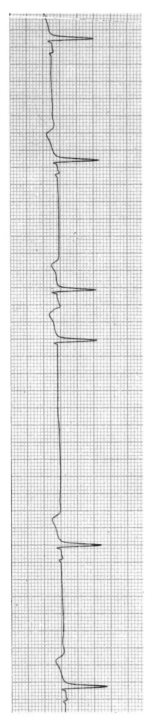

*Fig.* 3.3. The third ventricular complex is a junctional escape beat which arises after a period of sinus arrest. The escape beat is followed by an atrial ectopic beat which is superimposed on the preceding T wave and is conducted with a prolonged PR interval.

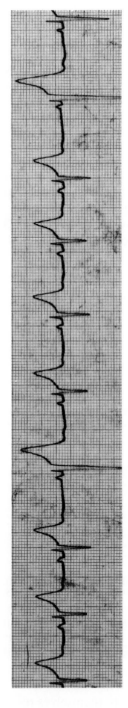

*Fig.* 3.4. The fourth and ninth ventricular complexes are escape beats, probably arising from the ventricles, which result from slowing of the sinus node rate. P waves precede the escape beats but it is unlikely that they have captured the ventricles since the PR intervals are shorter than during sinus rhythm.

## Main Points

1. The coupling interval of escape beats is greater than the cycle length of the dominant rhythm.

2. As with ectopic beats, the configuration of escape beats indicates whether they are of supraventricular or ventricular origin.

3. In contrast to ectopic beats, escape beats should never be suppressed by drugs.

# Chapter 4

# Bundle Branch Blocks

The bundle of His divides into left and right bundle branches. The left bundle branch has two main subdivisions: the anterior and posterior fascicles.

## RIGHT BUNDLE BRANCH BLOCK

In right bundle branch block, activation of the right ventricle is delayed. Septal and left ventricular activation are unaffected.

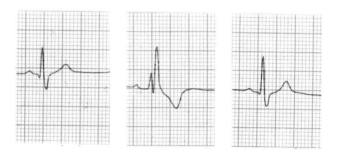

*Fig.* 4.1. Right bundle branch block (leads I, V1, V6). There is an M-shaped complex in V1 and a deep slurred S wave in leads I and V6.

Delayed right ventricular activation is reflected by an increase in duration of the QRS complex ($\geqslant 0.12$ s), a secondary R wave in leads orientated to the right ventricle (V1 and V2) and a slurred S wave in left ventricular leads, especially lead I (*Fig.* 4.1).

Partial right bundle branch block gives rise to a similar ECG appearance but the QRS duration is 0·11 s or less.

### Causes

Right bundle branch block may be an isolated congenital lesion. It is frequently found in congenital heart disease and other causes of right ventricular hypertrophy or strain.

Right bundle branch block is common when there is disease of the specialized conducting tissues. Phasic aberrant intraventricular conduction may cause intermittent right bundle branch block.

Based on limited data, neither pre-existing or acquired right bundle branch block appear to be of poor prognostic significance.

## LEFT BUNDLE BRANCH BLOCK

In left bundle branch block, activation of the interventricular septum is initiated by impulses arising from the right bundle branch and is therefore in the opposite direction to normal. Thus, the initial small negative (q)

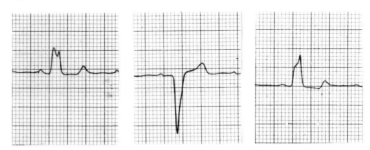

*Fig.* 4.2. Left bundle branch block (leads I, V1, V6). There is an M-shaped complex in I and V6. The QS complex in V1 is also characteristic of left bundle branch block.

wave normally seen in left ventricular leads (V5, V6, I and AVL) is replaced by a larger positive (R) wave. Activation of the left ventricle will be delayed and this results in a secondary R wave in left ventricular leads and prolongation of the duration of the QRS complex ($\geqslant 0.12$ s). The primary and secondary R waves produce an M-shaped ventricular complex in left ventricular leads (*Fig.* 4.2). In contrast, right bundle branch block produces an M-shaped ventricular complex in right ventricular leads.

Partial left bundle branch block has a similar ECG appearance to complete left bundle branch block, but the QRS duration is 0.10 or 0.11 s.

### Causes

Causes include coronary artery disease, severe left ventricular hypertrophy and cardiomyopathy. Rarely, left bundle branch block may occur in an otherwise normal heart. In this situation the block is often intermittent, there being anteroseptal T wave inversion when bundle branch block is absent (*Fig.* 4.3).

Like right bundle branch block, left bundle branch block can be due to disease of the specialized conduction tissues. It can also occur as a result of phasic aberrant intraventricular conduction.

The finding of recently acquired left bundle branch block indicates that the patient is at a substantially increased risk of sudden death.

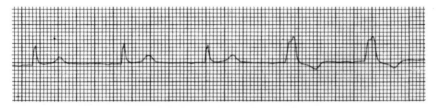

*Fig.* 4.3. Intermittent left bundle branch block (lead AVL).

## LEFT ANTERIOR AND POSTERIOR FASCICULAR BLOCKS

The anterior and posterior fascicles of the left bundle branch conduct impulses to the anterosuperior and posteroinferior regions of the left ventricle, respectively.

Block can occur in either the anterior or posterior fascicle and is known as fascicular block or hemiblock. Explanation of the diagnosis of the fascicular blocks is based on the hexaxial reference system.

### Hexaxial Reference System

Whereas the chest leads reflect electrical activity in the horizontal plane, the limb leads reflect activity in the frontal plane. The hexaxial reference system is a method of displaying the orientation of the six limb leads to the heart in the frontal plane (*Fig.* 4.4).

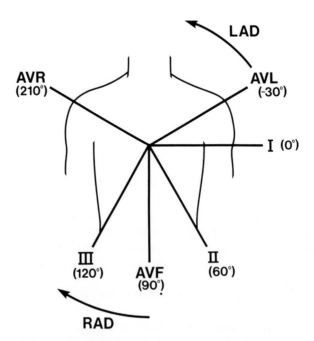

*Fig.* 4.4. Hexaxial reference system. LAD, left axis deviation; RAD, right axis deviation.

For example, a superiorly directed impulse will move away from leads II, III and AVF, producing a negative wave in these leads, and towards AVL, producing a positive wave in this lead.

The direction of an impulse can be expressed in terms of the number of degrees clockwise (positive) or anticlockwise (negative) of lead I, which is the zero reference point. For example, an impulse directed towards lead AVL has an axis of $-30°$ and an impulse directed towards lead III has an axis of $+120°$ (*Fig.* 4.4).

## Mean Frontal QRS Axis

The mean frontal QRS axis describes the dominant or average direction of the various electrical forces that develop during ventricular activation. Normally, the mean frontal QRS axis lies between AVL (i.e. $-30°$) and AVF (i.e. $+90°$). If the axis is counterclockwise, or to the left of AVL (i.e. less than $-30°$), it is termed abnormal left axis deviation. If the axis is clockwise, or to the right of AVF (i.e. more than $+90°$), there is right axis deviation.

Using the hexaxial reference system, it is possible to calculate the mean frontal QRS axis to within a few degrees. From the practical point of view, however, this degree of precision is unnecessary. Furthermore, though the method for calculating the axis is straightforward, errors are often made, sometimes leading to inappropriate action, e.g. unnecessary pacemaker insertion. It is easier and quite proper to diagnose left and right axis deviation from a simple rule of thumb, as follows.

In left axis deviation, lead I is predominantly positive and both leads II and III are predominantly negative (*Fig.* 4.5). Contrary to some older texts, *both* II and III must be predominantly negative, i.e. if in lead II the S wave is smaller than the R wave, left axis deviation is not present (*Fig.* 4.6). If lead II is equiphasic, there is borderline left axis deviation (*Fig.* 4.6). In right axis deviation lead I is predominantly negative and both leads II and III are predominantly positive (*Fig.* 4.7).

## LEFT ANTERIOR FASCICULAR BLOCK

Block in the anterior fascicle of the left bundle branch causes delay in activation of the anterosuperior portion of the left ventricle, whilst activation of the posteroinferior portion is unaffected.

Initial left ventricular activation will be via the posterior fascicle to the posteroinferior region and will therefore be directed inferiorly and to the right. This results in an initial positive deflection (r wave) in inferiorly orientated leads (II, III and AVF) and in an initial negative deflection (q wave) in the lateral leads (I and AVL) (*Fig.* 4.5).

The anterosuperior region will be activated by conduction from the posteroinferior region. The resultant wave will, therefore, be superiorly directed (R wave in I and AVL, S in II, III and AVF). Because conduction

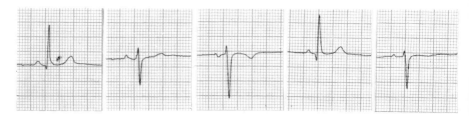

*Fig.* 4.5. Left axis deviation due to left anterior fascicular block (leads I, II, III, AVL, AVF).

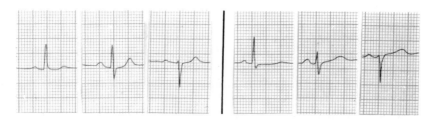

*Fig.* 4.6. Leads I, II, III from two patients. In the first, the mean frontal QRS axis is normal. In the second, lead II is equiphasic and thus there is borderline left axis deviation.

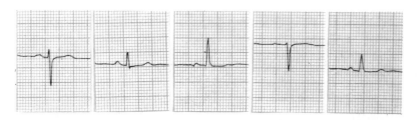

*Fig.* 4.7. Right axis deviation due to left posterior fascicular block (leads I, II, III, AVL, AVF).

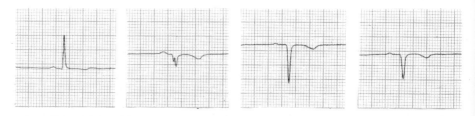

*Fig.* 4.8. Inferior myocardial infarction (leads I, II, III, AVF). There is left axis deviation but not left anterior fascicular block.

is through ordinary myocardium rather than the specialized conducting tissues, it will be relatively slow. As a result, activation of the antero-superior region will be delayed and consequently unopposed by activity from the rest of the ventricles. Thus, the resultant superiorly directed wave is larger than the initial inferiorly directed wave and the mean frontal QRS axis will also be superiorly directed, i.e. there will be left axis deviation.

Left anterior fascicular block is a common cause of left axis deviation. There are other causes, however; inferior myocardial infarction (*Fig.* 4.8) for example. To diagnose left anterior fascicular block two criteria must be satisfied. First, there must be left axis deviation, i.e. lead I must be predominantly positive and leads II and III predominantly negative. Secondly, the initial direction of ventricular activation must be inferior and to the right, i.e. there must be an initial r wave in leads II, III and AVF.

## LEFT POSTERIOR FASCICULAR BLOCK

In left posterior fascicular block activation of the posteroinferior portion of the left ventricle is delayed. As a result, there will be an initial positive (r) wave in leads I and AVL and an initial negative (q) wave in leads II, III and AVF; and there will be right axis deviation, i.e. lead I will be predominantly negative and leads II and III predominantly positive (*Fig.* 4.7).

A diagnosis of left posterior fascicular block can only be made in the absence of other causes of right axis deviation, i.e. any cause of right ventricular hypertrophy or strain, or a young patient with an asthenic build.

Left anterior and posterior fascicular blocks are commonly seen in conduction tissue disease. Their significance is discussed in Chapter 9.

## Main Points

1. Complete bundle branch block prolongs QRS duration to 0·12 s or greater. In incomplete block QRS duration is 0·10–0·11 s.

2. In left axis deviation, lead I is predominantly positive and leads II and III are predominantly negative.

3. In right axis deviation, lead I is predominantly negative and leads II and III positive.

4. The criteria for left anterior hemiblock are left axis deviation together with a small, initial r wave in leads II and AVF.

5. Left posterior hemiblock should be considered when there is right axis deviation in the absence of its other causes, e.g. right ventricular hypertrophy or strain.

*Chapter* **5**

# Ventricular
# Tachycardia

Ventricular tachycardia is defined as three or more ventricular ectopic beats in rapid succession. The rate is usually between 120 and 250 beats/min. A similar rhythm with a rate below 120/min is termed idioventricular tachycardia.

Ventricular tachycardia can cause shock, cardiac arrest or progress to ventricular fibrillation. On the other hand, some patients will have minor or even no symptoms.

The causes of ventricular tachycardia are:

Acute myocardial ischaemia and infarction
Chronic ischaemic heart disease
Hypertrophic cardiomyopathy
Congestive cardiomyopathy
Right ventricular dilated cardiomyopathy
Myocarditis
Mitral valve prolapse
Valvular heart disease
Drug toxicity, e.g. digoxin, quinidine
Hypokalemia
Hereditary prolongation of QT interval
Cardiac surgery
Uhl's syndrome
Idiopathic

## ECG Characteristics

The ventricular complexes are abnormal in shape and duration (*Fig.* 5.1). The duration of the ventricular complex is usually greater than 0·12 s,

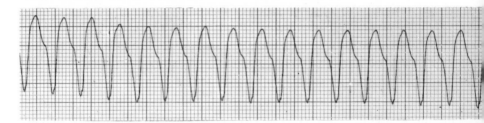

*Fig.* 5.1. Ventricular tachycardia. The complexes are broad and bizarre. The rhythm is regular.

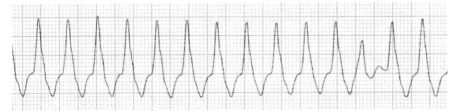

*Fig.* 5.2.  Ventricular tachycardia (lead V1). The right bundle branch block appearance to the complexes suggests a left ventricular origin. (The twelfth complex is a fusion beat, see below).

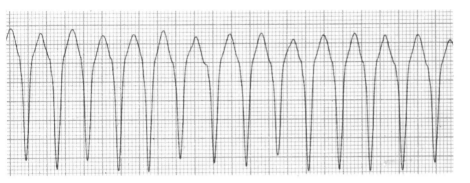

*Fig.* 5.3. Ventricular tachycardia (lead V1). The left bundle branch block appearance suggests a right ventricular origin.

although occasionally, when the focus is in the origin of the right or left bundle branches, thereby facilitating more rapid ventricular activation, it may be narrower.

The rhythm is regular unless there are capture beats (*see* below) which cause minor disturbances to the rhythm. An appearance of the complexes similar to right bundle branch block suggests a left ventricular origin of the tachycardia and vice versa (*Figs.* 5.2, 5.3).

### Atrial Activity During Ventricular Tachycardia

In 50 per cent of ventricular tachycardias atrial activity continues to be initiated by the sinus node and therefore proceeds independently of, and at a slower rate than, ventricular activity. In the other 50 per cent of such tachycardias the ventricular impulses are conducted via the AV junction to the atria so that each ventricular complex is followed by an inverted P wave (rarely second degree block may develop in the AV junction so that only a proportion of ventricular impulses are conducted to the atria). Often, the retrograde P wave is concealed by the superimposed terminal portion of the ventricular complex.

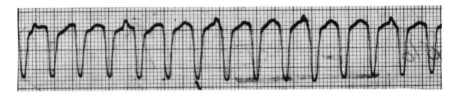

*Fig.* 5.4. Ventricular tachycardia with direct evidence of independent atrial activity. P waves, separated by intervals of 1·0 s, can be seen after the first, fourth, seventh, tenth and thirteenth ventricular complexes.

Identification of independent atrial activity during a tachycardia excludes an origin at AV node level or above and is thus an important sign in distinguishing between ventricular tachycardia and supraventricular tachycardia with phasic aberrant conduction (i.e. rate-related bundle branch block). There may be direct or only indirect evidence of independent atrial activity.

Direct evidence of independent atrial activity will be indicated by P waves inscribed at a slower rate than and dissociated from ventricular activity (*Fig.* 5.4). Inevitably, some P waves will be concealed by superimposed ventricular complexes, and not all leads will clearly show atrial activity. Thus a rhythm strip is often inadequate and a simultaneous recording of several ECG leads may be necessary. Sometimes there will be doubt as to whether small waves found on the ECG during tachycardia are actually P waves. If they are, they will be separated by similar intervals, or multiples of that interval.

There may, however, be only indirect evidence of independent atrial activity, i.e. capture or fusion beats. The finding of just one of these beats is sufficient to exclude an origin for the tachycardia above the level of the AV junction.

Capture beats occur when the timing of an atrial impulse during ventricular tachycardia is such that it can be transmitted via the AV junction and activate the ventricles before the next discharge from the ventricular focus. This results in a normal and therefore narrower ventricular complex,

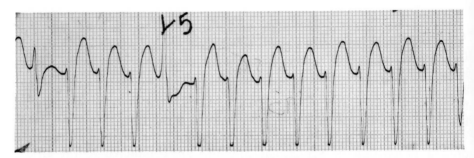

*Fig.* 5.5. Ventricular tachycardia (lead V5). The 'fifth complex is a capture beat and the first complex is a fusion beat.

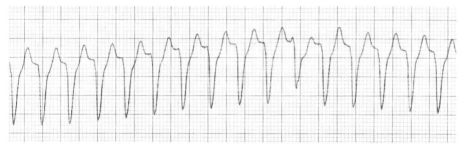

*Fig.* 5.6. Ventricular tachycardia. The eleventh complex is a fusion beat.

occurring slightly earlier than the next ventricular ectopic beat would be expected (*Fig.* 5.5).

Fusion beats are caused by a similar process. In this case, however, the ventricles are activated slightly later by the atrial impulse, resulting in simultaneous activation of the ventricles by both the transmitted atrial impulse and the ventricular ectopic focus. The result is a QRS complex which in appearance is a fusion between a normal QRS complex and a ventricular ectopic beat (*Figs.* 5.2, 5.5, 5.6).

## TREATMENT

Choice of treatment depends on the degree of circulatory disturbance caused by the tachycardia and whether the arrhythmia is likely to be a recurrent problem.

### Cardioversion

If ventricular tachycardia causes cardiac arrest or shock, immediate cardioversion is indicated (*see* Chapter 13). Cardioversion may also be indicated if anti-arrhythmic drugs are ineffective, contraindicated or cause haemodynamic deterioration without termination of the tachycardia. On the other hand, when ventricular tachycardia occurs in short, self-terminating episodes (*Fig.* 5.7) cardioversion is clearly inappropriate.

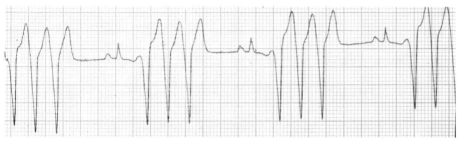

*Fig.* 5.7. Short, self-terminating episodes of ventricular tachycardia.

### Intravenous Anti-arrhythmic Drugs

For restoration of sinus rhythm, drugs are given intravenously. Lignocaine is the first-line drug. If this fails, mexiletine, disopyramide and flecainide are useful second-line drugs.

When frequently recurrent ventricular tachycardia is refractory to lignocaine or a second-line drug, amiodarone can be very effective in controlling the arrhythmia though it rarely has an immediate effect: unlike most drugs, it usually does not work 'at the end of a needle'.

All anti-arrhythmic drugs can, to varying degrees, impair myocardial performance and may therefore cause shock or heart failure. If these complications do occur, cardioversion should be quickly undertaken because return to sinus rhythm will usually improve cardiac output.

In general, no more than two anti-arrhythmic drugs should be given before considering another method of arrhythmia termination. In patients in heart failure or in whom extensive myocardial damage is suspected (e.g. a very large enzyme rise after infarction), drugs which can markedly impair myocardial action, e.g. disopyramide and flecainide, should be avoided or at least be given 'cautiously'.

Anti-arrhythmic drugs are discussed more fully in Chapter 12.

It is usual to follow a bolus of an intravenous drug with a continuous infusion because blood levels of most drugs fall rapidly after a single bolus. This makes good sense if it is anticipated that ventricular tachycardia may recur within a short period of time, e.g. in acute myocardial infarction or after cardiac surgery. It is pointless, however, to set up an infusion if either the bolus has failed to work or if the tachycardia is known to be an infrequent occurrence. In the latter case, the patient should be established on oral therapy.

### Oral Anti-arrhythmic Drugs

A number of oral anti-arrhythmic drugs may be useful for preventing a recurrence of ventricular tachycardia, e.g. quinidine, mexiletine, tocainide, disopyramide, flecainide and amiodarone. The latter two are the most effective.

Though it would seem logical to assume that the oral preparation of a drug, which when given intravenously has restored sinus rhythm, would be effective in preventing a recurrence of the arrhythmia, this is often not the case in practice. Whatever treatment is chosen, it is important to try to ensure that it is effective because a recurrence may be fatal.

Monitoring the electrocardiogram while in hospital, ambulatory ECG monitoring and exercise ECG testing are all useful and simple guides as to the efficacy of anti-arrhythmic therapy. Some also advocate close attention to plasma drug levels and intracardiac electrophysiological testing, but the author feels these are of limited practical value.

## Pacing

Pacing can sometimes be successful in terminating ventricular tachycardia. It should be considered where drugs are ineffective, when frequent recurrence necessitates multiple cardioversions or when a pacing wire is already in place for treatment of a conduction disorder.

The usual method is rapid (overdrive) right ventricular pacing (*Fig. 5.8*). A burst lasting a few seconds at a rate 10–30 per cent in excess of the tachycardia often terminates the arrhythmia, although there is a risk of accelerating the tachycardia or of precipitating ventricular fibrillation. If ventricular fibrillation does occur it should not be regarded as a disaster since cardioversion may well have proved necessary anyway.

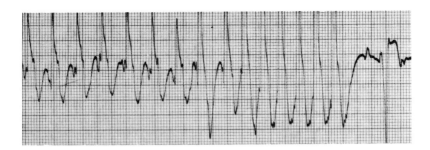

*Fig.* 5.8. Ventricular tachycardia (175/min) terminated by a brief period of overdrive ventricular pacing (225/min).

## Refractory Ventricular Tachycardias

Occasionally ventricular tachycardia cannot be controlled by even the most powerful of drugs. In these patients there are a number of newer methods of treatment, still undergoing development and evaluation, which might be of value.

Some ventricular tachycardias are due to a re-entrant mechanism and may be terminated by precisely timed single, double or even triple ventricular extrastimuli in the same way that AV re-entrant can be controlled. However, there is a risk of these stimuli initiating a more serious ventricular arrhythmia. Furthermore, unlike AV re-entrant tachycardia, the electrophysiological characteristics and response to pacing of a ventricular tachycardia can vary from time to time, so that long-term anti-tachycardia pacing is rarely undertaken and is unlikely to be trouble-free.

Methods for both temporary and long-term transvenous cardioversion have recently been developed. Much lower energy levels are required for shocks delivered by a transvenous lead as compared with transcutaneous cardioversion. A 'micro-shock' of sufficient energy will usually terminate ventricular tachycardia but micro-shocks can be painful and there are problems with implantable devices in distinguishing supraventricular from ventricular tachycardia. As with pacing, there is a risk that a micro-shock will actually accelerate the tachycardia.

Implantable defibrillators are also being evaluated. Improvements in technology may make them a practical proposition for difficult cases but currently the devices are very expensive and bulky, require thoracotomy for implantation, may not reliably recognize ventricular tachycardia or fibrillation and can provide only a limited number of shocks before having to be replaced.

A number of surgical techniques have been used to control ventricular tachycardia. These involve the excision or isolation of the arrhythmia focus. However, potential candidates for surgery often have impaired ventricular function. Cardiopulmonary bypass carries a substantial risk if ventricular function is poor and ventriculotomy may worsen ventricular function.

## IDIOVENTRICULAR TACHYCARDIA

This is defined as ventricular tachycardia with a rate less than 120/min (*Fig.* 5.9). It is usually seen in acute myocardial infarction. Treatment is unnecessary, although occasionally acceleration of the rate can occur and necessitate treatment.

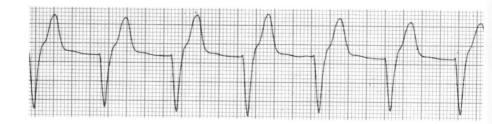

*Fig.* 5.9. Idioventricular tachycardia.

## TORSADE DE POINTES TACHYCARDIA

This is an atypical ventricular tachycardia, both in its ECG appearance and treatment. In contrast to the usual form of ventricular tachycardia, which consists of a rapid succession of extrasystoles which all have the same configuration, torsade de pointes is characterised by repeated progressive changes in the QRS axis so that the complexes appear to 'twist' about the baseline (*Fig.* 5.10). Its recognition is very important because it may be aggravated by anti-arrhythmic drugs and because correction of the underlying cause should prevent the arrhythmia.

The arrhythmia is caused by bradycardia and by drugs or disorders

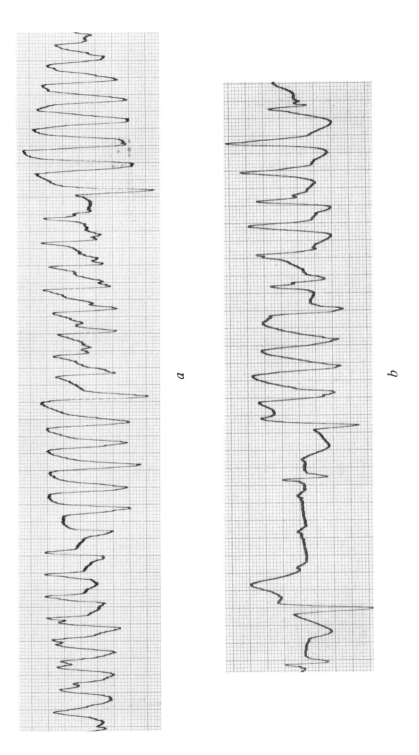

*Fig.* 5.10.  Two examples of torsade de pointes tachycardia: one (*a*) due to prenylamine and the other (*b*) caused by AV block.

that lead to abnormal ventricular repolarization, as set out below:

> Sick sinus syndrome
> AV block
> Anti-arrhythmic drugs
> Congenital QT interval prolongation
> Hypokalaemia
> Prenylamine
> Tricyclic antidepressants

Some patients have a long QT interval even without drugs. In these patients drugs such as quinidine and disopyramide, which can have a major effect on QT interval, should not be used in order to avoid precipitating torsade de pointes tachycardia. Toxic doses of anti-arrhythmic drugs, singly or in combination, can cause the arrhythmia. Increasing the heart rate by pacing will often prevent the tachycardia while the drug(s) are being excreted or metabolised.

## QT INTERVAL

The QT interval normally shortens with increasing heart rate, partly due to the increase in heart rate itself and partly due to the increase in sympathetic nervous system activity which is associated with a tachycardia. When measuring the QT interval it is necessary to correct it for heart rate with the following formula:

$$\text{Corrected QT interval (QT}_c) = \frac{\text{measured QT interval}}{\sqrt{\text{cycle length}}}.$$

The normal $QT_c$ should not exceed 0·42 s. It is reported that in some patients with hereditary prolongation of the QT interval, the interval either fails to shorten or actually increases as the heart rate rises with exercise.

### Congenital Prolongation of the QT Interval

There are two syndromes in which there is congenital prolongation of the QT interval (*Fig.* 5.11) and a tendency to ventricular tachycardia – the Jervell and Lange-Nielsen syndrome and the Romano–Ward syndrome.

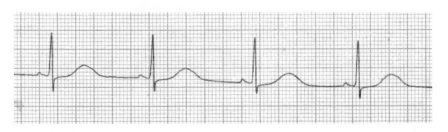

*Fig.* 5.11. QT interval prolongation. ($QT_c = 0·57$ s.)

The former is due to a recessive gene and is associated with nerve deafness, the latter is due to a dominant gene and is without deafness.

Ventricular tachycardia is usually induced by exertion or emotion and often causes syncope. Sudden death can occur and this may explain why most cases are seen in children or young adults.

The disorders are thought to be due to imbalance between left and right sympathetic innervation of the heart. Full beta-blockade is often effective in controlling symptoms. Occasionally, left cervical sympathectomy has been successful.

## Main Points

1. Ventricular tachycardia consists of a rapid, regular succession of ventricular extrasystoles. Normally, QRS duration exceeds 0·12 s.

2. There are many causes including ischaemic heart disease, cardiomyopathies and mitral valve prolapse.

3. The presence of P waves dissociated from ventricular activity or of fusion or capture beats indicates independent atrial activity and confirms a ventricular origin of the tachycardia.

4. If the tachycardia causes shock, cardioversion should be promptly carried out.

5. Lignocaine is the intravenous drug of choice. Generally, no more than two drugs should be tried before considering alternative methods of treatment.

6. Oral drugs may not prevent recurrence and ECG monitoring is essential in assessing their efficacy.

7. Idioventricular tachycardia is ventricular tachycardia at a rate less than 120 beats per minute. Treatment is not required.

8. Torsade de pointes tachycardia differs from the usual form of ventricular tachycardia in its ECG appearance, causes and treatment. Anti-arrhythmic drugs may aggravate the arrhythmia and pacing is often effective.

# Chapter 6

# Tachycardias of Supraventricular Origin

Several different types of tachycardia originate from the atria or AV junction:

Paroxysmal supraventricular (AV re-entrant) tachycardia
Atrial fibrillation
Atrial flutter
Atrial tachycardia
Junctional tachycardia
Sinus tachycardia (*see* Chapter 1)

It is important to appreciate that within this group of tachycardias there are major differences in mechanism, ECG characteristics and treatment.

The tachycardias have one thing in common: because they arise from above the level of the bundle branches, they usually result in narrow ventricular complexes. This has led some to use 'supraventricular tachycardia' as a blanket term for all the arrhythmias listed above. Others reserve the term for the type of arrhythmia illustrated in *Fig.* 6.1. The correct title for this arrhythmia is paroxysmal AV re-entrant tachycardia, but this term has not been widely adopted outside electrophysiological circles. Both its mechanism and response to drugs are different from other arrhythmias of supraventricular origin.

In this book 'tachycardias of supraventricular origin' will be used to cover the whole group and 'paroxysmal supraventricular tachycardia' will be reserved specifically for a tachycardia due to a re-entry mechanism involving the AV node (*Fig.* 6.1).

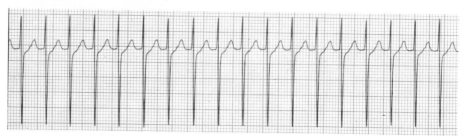

*Fig.* 6.1. Paroxysmal supraventricular tachycardia. It is due to a re-entry mechanism involving the AV node, hence the term AV re-entrant tachycardia.

# PAROXYSMAL SUPRAVENTRICULAR TACHYCARDIA

## Mechanism (*Fig.* 6.2)

In most cases the heart is structurally normal, i.e. there is no valve, myo-cardial or coronary disease. The arrhythmia is due to the repeated circu-lation of an impulse between atria and ventricles. It can only occur if there are two – rather than the usual one – connections between atria and ventricles. The additional connection either bypasses the AV node

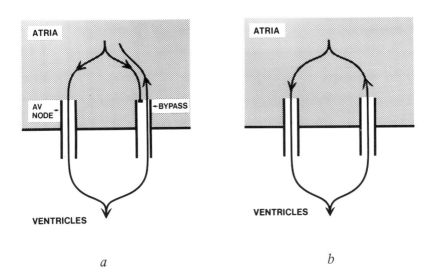

*a*                                                    *b*

*Fig.* 6.2. Initiation of AV re-entrant tachycardia. An atrial extrasystole arrives at the AV junction while the bypass tract is still refractory to excitation. The extrasystole is therefore only conducted to the ventricles via the AV node. By the time the extrasystole has traversed the AV node and reached the ventricles, the bypass tract has recovered and can conduct the impulse back to the atria (*a*) thereby initiating the re-entrant mechanism (*b*).

(pre-excitation syndromes, *see* Chapter 7) or is actually within, but functionally separate from, the AV node. The impulse is conducted from atria to ventricles by the normal AV junction and then re-enters the atria via the additional connection.

A variety of terms is used to refer to this arrhythmia. Some reflect its mechanism, e.g. AV nodal re-entrant tachycardia, AV junctional re-entrant tachycardia and reciprocating AV tachycardia, while others are inappropriate, e.g. atrial tachycardia and junctional tachycardia, because these terms are also used to refer to tachycardias due to enhanced automaticity. In this book 'paroxysmal supraventricular tachycardia' will be used instead of these terms.

### ECG Characteristics

The tachycardia is regular and unless there is pre-existing bundle branch block or phasic aberrant intraventricular conduction (i.e. bundle branch block caused by tachycardia), the QRS complexes are narrow (*Figs.* 6.1, 6.3–6.5). Normal P waves will not be seen during this arrhythmia though inverted P waves are sometimes identifiable within the ST segment of the ventricular complex (*Fig.* 7.8).

The rate during tachycardia can range from 130 to 250/min. In an individual patient the rate is fairly constant but is influences by sympathetic tone. For example, sympathetic activity and consequently the speed of AV nodal conduction may be increased by assuming a standing position with the result that the tachycardia becomes faster.

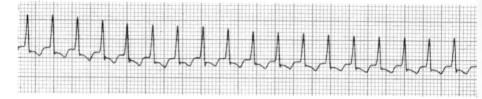

*Fig.* 6.3.   Paroxysmal supraventricular tachycardia.

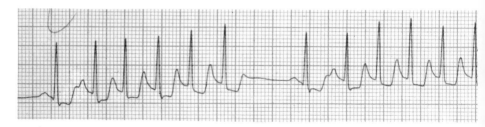

*Fig.* 6.4.   Initiation of paroxysmal supraventricular tachycardia. The first and seventh beats are of sinus node origin and are followed by atrial extrasystoles which initiate tachycardia (lead II).

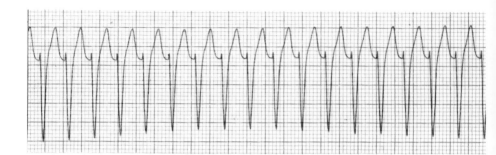

*Fig.* 6.5.   Paroxysmal supraventricular tachycardia with rate-related left bundle branch block (lead V1).

Since the circulating impulse re-enters the atria after ventricular activation, *each* QRS complex will be followed by an inverted P wave (*see* Chapter 7). If the atrial rate is seen to exceed the ventricular rate, whether spontaneously or due to a drug or manoeuvre which slows AV node conduction, then the rhythm is atrial tachycardia or flutter; paroxysmal supraventricular tachycardia is excluded.

As with most tachycardias, ST segment and T wave changes can be caused by the tachycardia and persist for some time after its cessation. The ST—T changes are of no diagnostic significance.

In patients with paroxysmal supraventricular tachycardia, the ECG during sinus rhythm is usually normal unless there is evidence of pre-excitation (*see* Chapter 7).

## Clinical Features

Paroxysmal supraventricular tachycardia is a common disorder. Attacks may start in infancy, childhood or adult life and are often recurrent. The duration and frequency of attacks are variable; they may last for a few minutes or for many hours, and may recur several times per day or be separated by many months.

The main symptom is rapid and often distressing palpitation of abrupt onset. Though the arrhythmia stops suddenly, not all patients are aware of this since sinus tachycardia often follows.

Faintness, syncope, polyuria and chest pain may also occur. Coexistent valvular, myocardial or coronary artery disease may lead to more serious problems. A very prolonged episode of tachycardia, even in a structurally normal heart, may cause heart failure.

## Treatment

Short episodes of tachycardia without distress do not require treatment.

### *Vagal Stimulation*

When termination of the tachycardia is indicated, the first approach should be vagal stimulation. By increasing vagal tone, AV node conduction may be slowed and the tachycardia circuit thereby interrupted. Carotid sinus massage is the best method. It is performed by digital pressure, using the first and second fingers, over the artery at the level of the upper border of the thyroid cartilage.

Other methods of vagal stimulation include the Valsalva manoeuvre, eyeball pressure, which is not recommended because it is extremely painful, and the 'diving reflex'. In the diving reflex the patient holds his breath and then immerses his face in ice-cold water. Stimulation of the

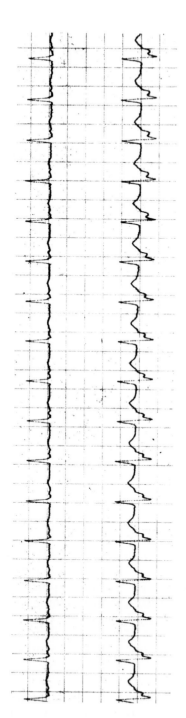

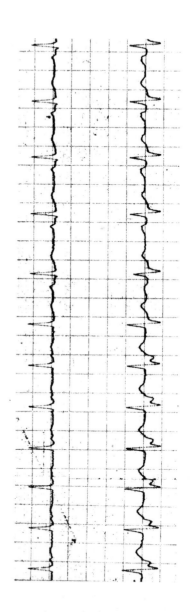

*Fig.* 6.6. Continuous trace: Paroxysmal supraventricular tachycardia slowed and then terminated by verapamil (leads I and II recorded simultaneously). There is a P wave immediately following each QRS complex, suggesting that the tachycardia is due to dual AV nodal pathways.

trigeminal nerves can cause an increase in vagal tone, particularly in the young. Occasionally, a short period of asystole may result. For obvious reasons, this procedure should not be carried out unsupervised.

## Intravenous Drugs

If vagal stimulation does not work, intravenous verapamil (5–10 mg over 30–60 s) will almost certainly terminate the arrhythmia within a couple of minutes (*Fig.* 6.6). Apparent failure of verapamil is usually due to giving too small a dose too slowly. If an adequate dose of verapamil fails to work, the diagnosis should be reconsidered! If the ventricular rate falls but sinus rhythm does not return, it is probable that the rhythm is atrial flutter or fibrillation. If there is no response, ventricular tachycardia is a possibility.

Verapamil must not be used if the patient has recently received an oral or intravenous beta-blocking drug (*see* Chapter 12). Beta-blockers are not as effective as verapamil, and since they preclude use of the latter they should not be employed as first-line treatment. Not infrequently, patients with paroxysmal supraventricular tachycardia are receiving oral beta-blockers. In this case an intravenous beta-blocking drug (e.g. practolol 5–10 mg, atenolol 5 mg or sotalol 20–60 mg) should be tried.

Other drugs such as digoxin, disopyramide and procainamide may also be effective (*see* Chapter 12). Digoxin does have the advantage of not being negatively inotropic. Disopyramide and procainamide affect conduction in the additional AV connection rather than the AV node.

## Electrical Methods

If drugs are ineffective or if clinical circumstances necessitate an immediate return to sinus rhythm, cardioversion should be carried out (*see* Chapter 13).

Various pacing methods can be used to terminate paroxysmal supraventricular tachycardia. The simplest of these is pacing the right atrium at a rate 20–30 per cent faster than the tachycardia (overdrive pacing). On abrupt termination of pacing, sinus rhythm will often return: if unsuccessful, pacing should be repeated several times (*Fig.* 6.7). There is a small risk of precipitating atrial fibrillation which usually will not last for many minutes before sinus rhythm is restored. However, in patients with Wolff–Parkinson–White syndrome atrial fibrillation might lead to a very fast ventricular response (Chapter 7). Fixed rate right ventricular pacing at 70–100/min (underdrive pacing) is sometimes effective (*Fig.* 6.7). More sophisticated and efficient pacing methods of tachycardia termination require the use of a programmable pacemaker which enables the introduction of a single or a couplet of precisely timed atrial or ventricular extrastimuli (*Fig.* 6.7). These pacing methods can be used on a long

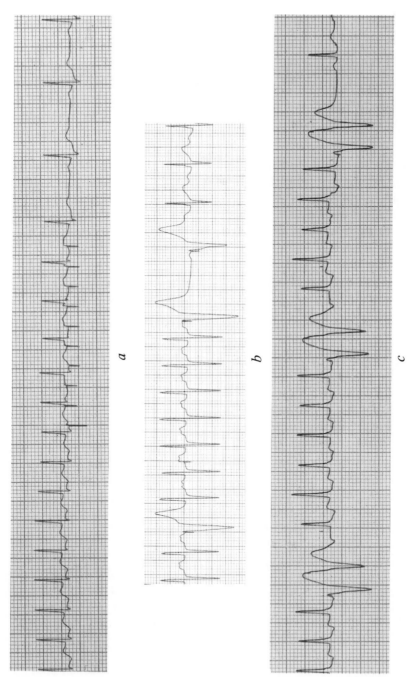

*Fig.* 6.7.   Three pacing methods of termination of AV re-entrant tachycardia. *a* Rapid atrial pacing. *b* Right ventricular underdrive pacing; the second pacing stimulus which captures the ventricles terminates the arrhythmia; *c* A scanning implanted pacemaker which introduces a couplet of precisely timed ventricular extrastimuli when tachycardia is detected. After every four cycles, the pacemaker introduces further couplets of extrastimuli 6 ms earlier in the cardiac cycle until sinus rhythm is restored.

term basis by implanting a pacemaker. Detailed intracardiac electrophysiological studies are necessary to assess suitability of long term
pacing.

## Prophylaxis

The patient should be reassured that the tachycardia is distressing rather
than dangerous and that it is due to an electrical rather than structural
cardiac abnormality.

A number of drugs may be of prophylactic value, including beta-
blockers (especially sotalol), digoxin, verapamil, disopyramide and
quinidine. Selection of a drug which is both effective and well tolerated
is often a process of trial and error. The author usually tries sotalol
(160–320 mg daily) first (*see* Chapter 12). Amiodarone is likely to be
effective in cases where other drugs have failed, but should be reserved
for refractory cases where the need for tachycardia control outweighs
the drug's possible unwanted effects. The patient should keep a record of
the number and duration of any attacks so that the effect of therapy can
be assessed.

In some patients, both drugs and anti-tachycardia pacing are ineffective.
An alternative is surgical division of one part of the re-entrant circuit: the
AV junction or, if accessible, the additional connection. Recently, non-
surgical ablation of AV conduction has been introduced. This is achieved
by passing a high energy (200–400 J) direct current shock to the AV
junction via a transvenous pacing lead positioned as close to the bundle
of His as possible (*Fig.* 6.8). In spite of the high energy used, damage is
confined to the region of the AV junction and the technique has proved
safe.

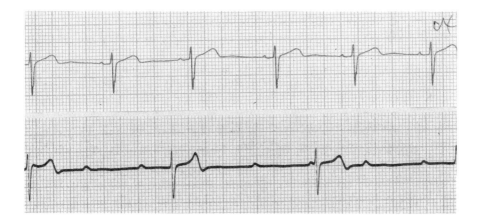

*Fig.* 6.8. Patient with paroxysmal supraventricular tachycardia before (upper trace) and after
(lower trace) transvenous AV nodal ablation.

Creation of heart block does necessitate pacemaker implantation. In most patients who have undergone transvenous ablation, it is necessary to implant a physiological pacemaker which will allow the heart rate to accelerate during exertion: a simple ventricular demand pacemaker will often lead to a markedly restricted exercise tolerance.

A similar technique has been used in a few patients for ablation of accessory pathways and foci of origin of atrial and ventricular tachycardias.

A detailed intracardial electrophysiological study is required to assess the feasibility of ablation, anti-tachycardia pacing and surgery.

## ENHANCED AUTOMATICITY

As a result of disease, or in some cases digoxin toxicity, a focus in the atria or AV junction can acquire enhanced automaticity and thereby discharge at a rate in excess of that of the sinus node and take control of the heart rhythm. This is thought to be the mechanism of atrial tachycardia, flutter and fibrillation, and also of junctional tachycardia. (It has been suggested that 'enhanced automaticity' may in fact be due to a re-entrant circuit involving only a few cells, but this is not of practical importance.)

Unlike paroxysmal supraventricular tachycardia, which is due to an AV node re-entrant circuit, supraventricular arrhythmias due to enhanced automaticity can not be expected to be terminated by drugs which slow AV nodal conduction. The drugs should, however, reduce the ventricular rate during the arrhythmia. Often with these arrhythmias the purpose of drug therapy is not to achieve a return to sinus rhythm but to control the ventricular response to the ectopic atrial focus.

## ATRIAL FIBRILLATION

In atrial fibrillation the atria discharge at a rate between 350 and 600/min. In the same way that ventricular fibrillation is usually initiated by a ventricular ectopic beat falling on the T wave of the preceding beat, atrial fibrillation is initiated by an atrial ectopic beat falling during the atrial recovery period (*Fig.* 6.9). Fortunately the AV node cannot conduct at a sufficient frequency to allow all atrial impulses to reach the ventricles. After an impulse has been conducted to the ventricles, the AV node will be refractory to excitation by other impulses for a short period. Some impulses only partially penetrate the AV node. They will not, therefore, activate the ventricles but do block or delay succeeding impulses. This process of 'concealed conduction' is responsible for the totally irregular ventricular response characteristic of atrial fibrillation.

Usually the AV node does not allow a ventricular rate in excess of 200/min, and when AV node conduction is depressed by drugs or disease the ventricular response will be much slower.

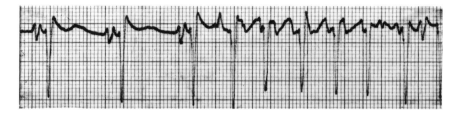

*Fig.* 6.9. Atrial fibrillation is initiated by an atrial ectopic beat superimposed on the ST segment of the third sinus beat.

## ECG Characteristics

The rapid and chaotic atrial activity is reflected by 'f' waves which are inscribed at a rate of 350–600/min and are irregular both in rate and size. However, particularly in longstanding cases of atrial fibrillation, f waves may not be seen in all ECG leads. They are usually best seen in lead V1 (*Figs.* 6.10–6.14). Clearly, P waves will be absent.

The hallmark of atrial fibrillation is a totally irregular ventricular response. In the absence of P waves, even if f waves are not seen, a completely irregular ventricular rate is diagnostic of atrial fibrillation. Atrial fibrillation with a rapid ventricular response is often misdiagnosed (*Figs.* 6.15, 6.16). If the characteristic irregular ventricular rate is remembered, this mistake will not be made.

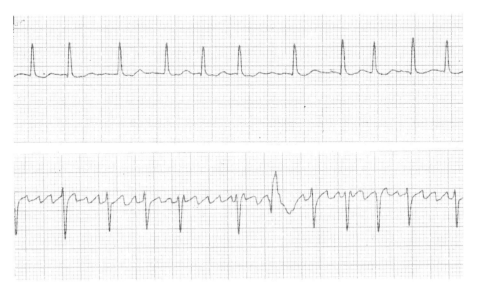

*Fig.* 6.10. Atrial fibrillation (leads 1 and V1). The ventricular rate is irregularly irregular and there are no P waves. 'f' waves are best seen in lead V1. (There is phasic aberrant conduction of the seventh QRS complex in V1.)

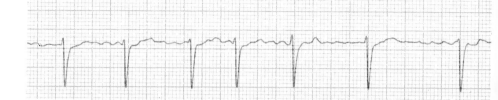

*Fig.* 6.11.  Atrial fibrillation (lead V1).

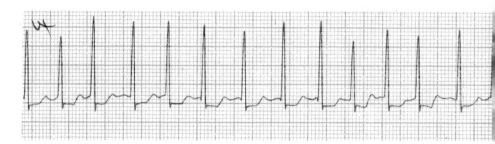

*Fig.* 6.12.  Atrial fibrillation. 'f' waves are not seen in this lead but the ventricular rate is totally irregular and there are no P waves.

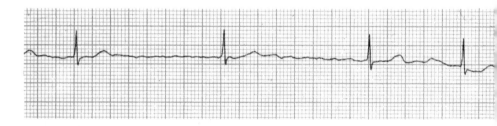

*Fig.* 6.13.  Atrial fibrillation with a slow ventricular response.

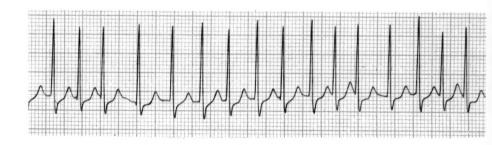

*Fig.* 6.14.  Atrial fibrillation with rapid ventricular response.

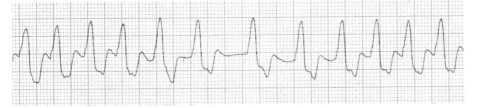

*Fig.* 6.15. Atrial fibrillation with broad ventricular complexes due to pre-existent left bundle branch block (lead V6).

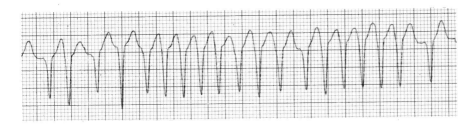

*Fig.* 6.16. Atrial fibrillation in a patient with Wolff–Parkinson–White syndrome. The bundle of Kent facilitates very frequent conduction of atrial impulses to the ventricles and causes broad ventricular complexes due to delta waves.

The only circumstance in which there will be a regular ventricular rhythm during atrial fibrillation is when it is complicated by complete AV block (*Fig.* 6.17).

Sometimes the pattern of atrial activity is so coarse that atrial flutter rather than fibrillation is suspected. In the latter case the atrial rate will usually be greater than 350/min and the ventricular response will be totally irregular (*Fig.* 6.18).

Phasic aberrant intraventricular conduction is often seen during atrial fibrillation. Aberration is the result of unequal recovery periods of the bundle branches. An early supraventricular impulse may reach the ventricles when one bundle branch is still refractory and therefore not capable of conduction whilst the other bundle branch has recovered and will conduct. The resultant ventricular complex will show bundle branch block. The right bundle usually has a longer refractory period than the left and, thus, right bundle branch block is more common. Refractory periods are prolonged with increasing cycle length. Thus, aberration is usually seen when a beat having a short cycle length follows one with a long cycle length (*Fig.* 6.19).

## Clinical features

Atrial fibrillation is one of the most common arrhythmias. Unlike AV re-entrant tachycardia, atrial fibrillation is often associated with other disease processes, cardiac or non-cardiac, and a cause should be sought.

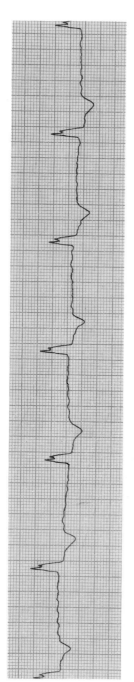

*Fig.* 6.17.   Atrial fibrillation with complete AV block. The ventricular rhythm is regular.

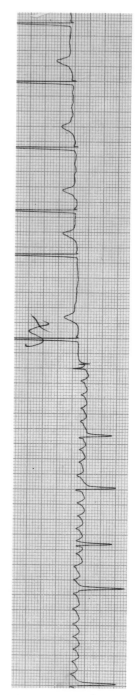

*Fig.* 6.18.   Atrial fibrillation. Continuous recording as the lead is changed from V1 to V4. There is a marked difference in baseline activity. The atrial rate is 375/min and the ventricular response is totally irregular.

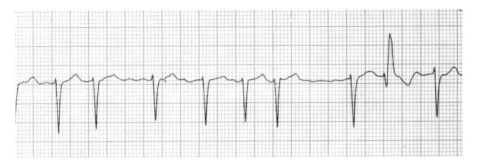

*Fig.* 6.19.  Atrial fibrillation (lead V1). The penultimate beat has a short cycle length and follows a beat with a long cycle length. It is conducted with right bundle branch block – phasic aberrant intraventricular conduction.

Causes include rheumatic heart disease, coronary and hypertensive heart disease, thyrotoxicosis, sick sinus syndrome, myopericarditis, dilated and hypertrophic cardiomyopathies, specific heart muscle diseases, constrictive pericarditis, atrial septal defect, alcohol abuse, pulmonary embolism, thoracotomy and trauma. In a substantial proportion of cases, the arrhythmia is idiopathic and is referred to as "lone atrial fibrillation".

Atrial fibrillation may be paroxysmal or persistent. The major determinant of prognosis is the presence or absence of organic heart disease. Paroxysmal lone atrial fibrillation has a normal prognosis.

During atrial fibrillation, stasis of blood in the left atrium may occur and lead to thrombus formation and systemic embolism. Patients with rheumatic mitral valve disease are at greatest risk whereas embolism is very rare in lone atrial fibrillation. In patients with atrial fibrillation from all causes except mitral valve disease, there is a five-fold increase in the incidence of stroke, whereas mitral valve disease increases the incidence to seventeen-fold. Several studies report a high incidence of systemic embolism in atrial fibrillation caused by acute thyrotoxicosis.

## Treatment

In most cases, treatment is aimed at controlling the ventricular response to atrial fibrillation by the use of a drug or drugs which depress AV nodal conduction. Although cardioversion will often restore sinus rhythm, there is a high relapse rate, particularly when there is cardiomegaly, marked left atrial enlargement, or when the arrhythmia has been present for a long time. Long-term quinidine, disopyramide or amiodarone do slightly reduce the relapse rate. When atrial fibrillation has been caused by an acute event, there is a good chance that sinus rhythm will be maintained after cardioversion.

Occasionally, atrial fibrillation with a rapid ventricular response will cause shock or severe heart failure and necessitate immediate cardio-version. When prompt reduction of the ventricular rate is required, digoxin or verapamil can be given intravenously: the latter will work within a couple of minutes. If there is no urgency, control can usually be achieved with oral digoxin. If control is unsatisfactory in spite of apparently adequate digitilization, the addition of verapamil (usually 40 mg t.d.s.) or a beta-blocker will effect control. Occasionally, these measures fail, in which case one may have to resort to amiodarone or even transvenous ablation of the AV junction. In patients with paroxysmal atrial fibrillation, suppression of atrial extrasytoles by quinidine or amio-darone may prevent further attacks.

Anticoagulation to prevent systemic embolism is indicated in cases of rheumatic mitral valve disease and when there is a history of embolism. It should also be considered in the bradycardia-tachycardia syndrome if tachyarrhythmias persist in spite of pacing (*see* Chapter 10), and in acute thyrotoxicosis.

## ATRIAL FLUTTER

Atrial flutter is less common than atrial fibrillation but the causes are the same. In atrial flutter the atria discharge at a rate between 250 and 350/min. In most cases the atrial rate is very close to 300/min.

Very rarely the AV node conducts all atrial impulses to the ventricles, resulting in a ventricular rate of 300/min. In most cases a degree of AV block occurs. In patients with a healthy AV note who are not receiving AV nodal-blocking drugs, it is usually 2 : 1 AV block.

### ECG Characteristics

The rapid atrial activity is reflected by 'F' waves which are regular. Often there is no isoelectric line between F waves so that the baseline has a 'saw-tooth' appearance. Though commonly seen, it is not essential for the diagnosis of atrial flutter. Sometimes, some ECG leads will show the saw-tooth appearance whilst others, particularly V1, will show discrete F waves (*Fig*. 6.20).

When there is a high degree of AV block, atrial flutter is easy to diagnose (*Fig*. 6.21). However, when there is 2 : 1 AV block, the rapid ventricular response may conceal atrial activity, with the result that the diagnosis of atrial flutter is frequently missed, often being mistaken for sinus tachycardia. The atrial rate in flutter is usually 300/min, and thus during 2 : 1 AV block the resultant ventricular rate will be 150/min. If this heart rate is found in a patient at rest, it should be assumed to be atrial flutter

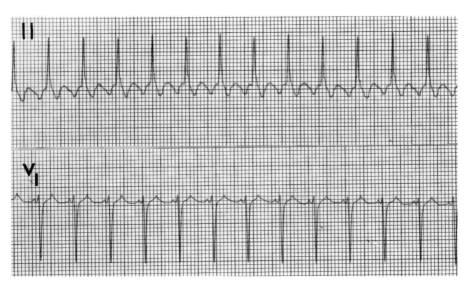

*Fig.* 6.20.  Atrial flutter with 2:1 AV block. Lead II shows a classic saw-tooth appearance whilst V1 shows discrete atrial waves. In V1 each QRS complex is immediately preceded by an F wave and is followed by an F wave which is superimposed on the T wave.

CSM

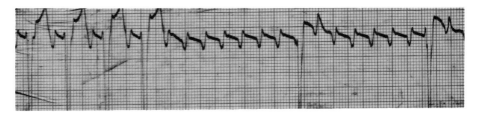

*Fig.* 6.21.  Atrial flutter with 2:1 AV block. The degree of AV block increases markedly with carotid sinus massage (CSM).

until proved otherwise. The ECG, particularly lead V1, should be closely inspected for signs of F waves (*Figs.* 6.22–6.24). Often, alternate F waves will be superimposed on ventricular T waves. To confirm that there is an F wave superimposed on the T wave, the interval between the atrial wave preceding the QRS complex and the peak on the T wave must be precisely the same as the interval between the T wave peak and the subsequent atrial wave. Carotid sinus massage (*Fig.* 6.21), or even intravenous verapamil, may be required to temporarily increase the degree of AV block for diagnostic purposes.

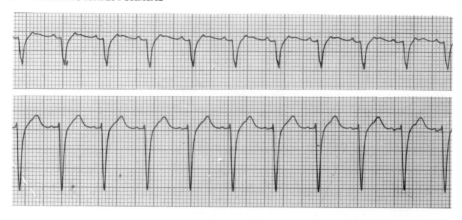

*Fig.* 6.22. Simultaneous recording of leads V1 and V2. Atrial flutter can be readily diagnosed from V1 (alternate F waves are superimposed on the beginning of the ventricular T wave) but V2 looks like sinus tachycardia.

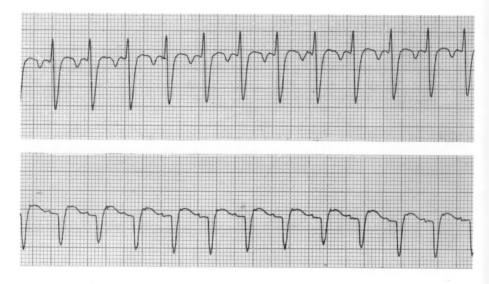

*Fig.* 6.23. Atrial flutter leads AVF and V1). AVF suggests a saw-tooth appearance, V1 shows discrete atrial activity at 300/min: alternate F waves are superimposed on the junction between the QRS complex and T wave.

When 1 : 1 AV conduction occurs the ventricular rate will be 300/min. This rate should also be assumed to be due to atrial flutter unless proved otherwise (*Fig.* 6.24).

As with atrial fibrillation, phasic aberrant intraventricular conduction can occur.

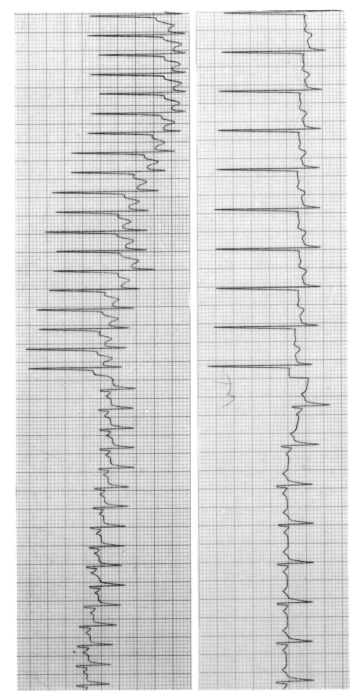

*Fig.* 6.24. Continuous recordings of leads V1 and V4. In the upper trace the ventricular rate is 300/min, suggesting atrial flutter with 1 : 1 AV conduction. The lower trace shows the effect of carotid sinus massage. The rate is halved and F waves can be seen, in V1, immediately preceding the QRS complex and superimposed on the T wave.

## Treatment

Unlike in atrial fibrillation, it is often difficult to control the ventricular rate during atrial flutter with AV nodal-blocking drugs. For this reason, if possible, a return to sinus rhythm should be sought.

Atrial flutter can almost always be terminated by cardioversion. Usually, a single low energy shock is sufficient. Initially the energy setting should be set at 25 watt-seconds (joules). If unsuccessful, 50 and then 100 Ws should be tried.

An alternative to cardioversion is rapid right atrial pacing. This has the advantages that general anaesthesia is not required and that it can be used repeatedly if atrial flutter is a frequently recurrent problem. The necessary pacing rate is usually 10–30 per cent in excess of the atrial rate and should be applied for 10–30 s. On abrupt cessation of pacing, sinus rhythm will return, after a short pause, in approximately one-third of patients. In another third, atrial fibrillation will be precipitated but this often spontaneously reverts to sinus rhythm over the next few hours. In one-third of cases the rhythm will be unchanged by atrial pacing. It is important to ensure that the pacing stimuli are capturing the atria and this is usually reflected by a change in ventricular rate during pacing.

Atrial flutter may occur in the sick sinus syndrome. When this is suspected, because of the risk of asystole, a temporary pacing electrode should be inserted prior to cardioversion.

In patients with a rapid ventricular rate, intravenous verapamil can be used to increase the degree of AV block temporarily. In about one-fifth of cases verapamil will actually restore sinus rhythm.

In patients with chronic atrial flutter in whom cardioversion has either been unsuccessful or contraindicated, AV nodal blocking drugs are usually required to control the ventricular response unless there is a high degree of AV block. Digoxin should be the initial choice, but it may be necessary to add verapamil. If this combination does not control the ventricular rate, substitution of amiodarone can be very effective: it usually slows both the atrial rate and the ventricular response.

It should be noted that in a few patients with atrial flutter and 2 : 1 AV block, the increased sympathetic nervous system activity associated with exercise may enhance AV conduction and result in 1 : 1 conduction and thus a ventricular rate of 300/min. Patients in this situation may experience near-syncope or syncope on exertion.


## ATRIAL TACHYCARDIA

The main difference between atrial tachycardia and flutter is that in the former the atrial rate is slower, being between 120 and 250/min. Again, sometimes the AV node can conduct all atrial impulses but often there is a degree of AV block. (With fairly high grades of AV block, because the atrial rate is relatively slow, the rhythm may be misdiagnosed as complete heart block (*Fig.* 6.25) and an inappropriate request made for cardiac pacing.)

## ECG Characteristics

Because the atrial rate is slower, there is no saw-tooth appearance to the baseline. Abnormally shaped P waves are inscribed at a regular rate (*Fig.* 6.25). Usually, the ventricular complexes will be narrow unless there is pre-existent bundle branch block or phasic aberrant intraventricular conduction.

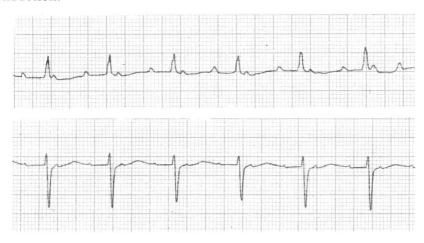

*Fig.* 6.25.  Atrial tachycardia with 2:1 AV block (leads AVF and V1). Atrial rate is 175/min.

Occasionally atrial tachycardia with 1 : 1 AV conduction occurs. As in atrial flutter, carotid sinus massage is often helpful in the diagnosis. Again like atrial flutter, atrial activity is often best seen in lead V1.

## Causes

Atrial tachycardia with AV block is commonly due to digoxin toxicity (*Fig.* 6.26). The arrhythmia is often referred to as 'paroxysmal atrial tachycardia with block', being abbreviated to PATB. The term paroxysmal is inappropriate; particularly in the context of digoxin toxicity, the arrhythmia is usually sustained.
    Other causes include cardiomyopathy, chronic ischaemic heart disease, rheumatic heart disease and sick sinus syndrome.

## Treatment

If the patient is receiving digoxin, toxicity should be suspected and the drug discontinued. When the patient has not had digoxin, this drug may

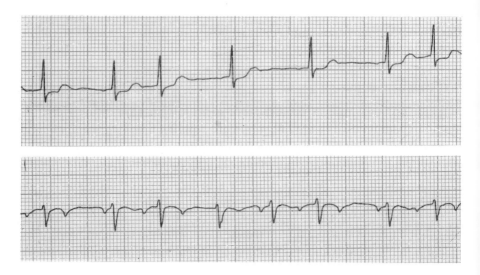

*Fig.* 6.26. Atrial tachycardia (leads II and V1) in a patient with digoxin toxicity. The limb lead suggested atrial fibrillation but V1 clearly shows atrial tachycardia with Mobitz type I AV block.

be used to control the ventricular rate.

If a return to sinus rhythm is required, cardioversion or rapid atrial pacing should be performed.

## JUNCTIONAL TACHYCARDIA

Junctional tachycardia is due to enhanced automaticity of the AV junction. It should be distinguished from paroxysmal supraventricular tachycardia which is due to a re-entry mechanism involving the AV node and which is sometimes inappropriately termed AV junctional tachycardia.

### ECG Characteristics

Usually the QRS complexes are similar to those during sinus rhythm and thus in most cases will be narrow. Occasionally the duration of the QRS complex is slightly longer than it would be during sinus rhythm (*Fig.* 6.27). Usually the junctional focus activates both atria and ventricles. Thus the QRS complex is either preceded by or succeeded by an inverted P wave. Sometimes retrograde atrial activation does not occur and then atrial activity will be independent of the junctional focus.

### Causes

Junctional tachycardia is commonly caused by digoxin toxicity. Most forms of cardiac disease, especially coronary artery disease, can also cause the arrhythmia.

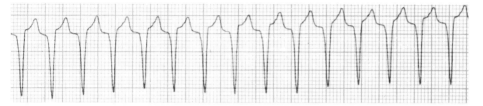

*Fig.* 6.27.  Junctional tachycardia (lead V2) in a patient with anterior myocardial infarction.

### Treatment

AV nodal blocking drugs may be effective. Otherwise, a drug which decreases automaticity of the focus, e.g. lignocaine or disopyramide, should be used. Where digoxin toxicity is suspected, the drug should be withdrawn.

## Main Points

**1.** There are several different tachycardias of supraventricular origin. For correct management of the patient, it is necessary to determine with which tachycardia one is dealing.

**2.** QRS duration during tachycardia will be normal unless there is pre-existing or rate-related bundle branch block.

**3.** Paroxysmal supraventricular (AV re-entrant) tachycardia requires the presence of a second electrical connection between atria and ventricles in addition to the AV node. Usually structural heart disease is absent. The ventricular rhythm is regular. Atrial activity is usually not seen but if found will be in the form of an inverted P wave after each QRS complex.

**4.** Atrial fibrillation, flutter and tachycardia are due to enhanced automaticity of atrial ectopic foci and are often associated with cardiac or extracardiac disease.

**5.** Atrial fibrillation is characterized by a totally irregular ventricular rhythm. Usually AV nodal-blocking drugs are used to control the ventricular response. Though cardioversion often restores sinus rhythm, there is a high relapse rate. Anticoagulation should be considered when the arrhythmia is associated with mitral valve disease, bradycardia-tachycardia syndrome and acute thyrotoxicosis.

**6.** The diagnosis of atrial flutter is based on the finding of atrial activity at a rate of approximately 300/min. Lead V1 is often the best lead for demonstrating atrial flutter: when there is 2 : 1 AV conduction, alternate F waves will be superimposed on ventricular T waves. Where possible, a return to sinus rhythm should be sought.

**7.** Atrial tachycardia is similar to flutter but the atrial rate is 120–250/min.

# Chapter 7

# Pre-excitation Syndromes

In the normal heart atrial impulses can only be conducted to the ventricles by the AV node. In the pre-excitation syndromes there is an additional connection between atria and ventricles. Unlike the AV node, the accessory connection does not delay conduction between atria and ventricles. Thus, atrial impulses will be transmitted more quickly by the accessory connection and will initiate ventricular activation before the atrial impulse has traversed the AV node; hence the term 'pre-excitation'.

## WOLFF–PARKINSON–WHITE SYNDROME

The syndrome is characterized by a short PR interval, a widened QRS complex due to the presence of a delta wave and a tendency to paroxysmal tachycardia.

Approximately 1·5/1000 of the population have the syndrome.

The Wolff–Parkinson–White syndrome is caused by an accessory connection between atrial and ventricular myocardium. This connection, which consists of ordinary myocardium, is referred to as an accessory AV pathway or bundle of Kent and is congenital in origin. Unlike tracts causing other pre-excitation syndromes, neither end of the connection is to any part of the specialized conducting system. The bundle of Kent may be situated anywhere in the AV groove.

### ECG Characteristics

Although an atrial impulse will be conducted more quickly by the bundle of Kent than by the normal AV node, once it has reached the ventricles further conduction is relatively slow because the bundle is connected to ordinary myocardium rather than specialized conducting tissues. This slow conduction is reflected by slurring of the ventricular complex, the delta wave (*Fig.* 7.1).

The syndrome is classified into types A and B, depending on the ventricular complex in lead V1. If predominantly positive, it is type A and if negative, type B (*Figs.* 7.2, 7.3). In type A syndrome the bundle of Kent is likely to be on the left side of the heart and in type B, on the right side. This rule, however, is not completely reliable.

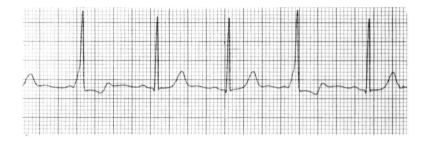

*Fig.* 7.1. Wolff–Parkinson–White syndrome. In this patient, the bundle of Kent conducts inter-mittently. The second, third and fifth complexes are normal whereas the first and fourth complexes show the characteristic short PR interval and delta wave. By comparing the pre-excited and normal beats, it can be seen how the delta wave both shortens the PR interval and broadens the ventricular complex.

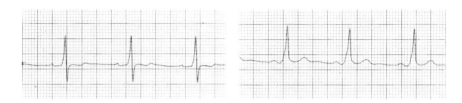

*Fig.* 7.2. Type A Wolff–Parkinson–White syndrome (leads V1 and V6).

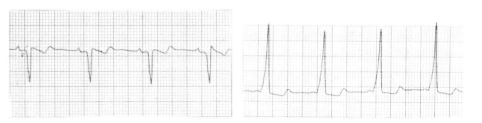

*Fig.* 7.3. Type B Wolff–Parkinson–White syndrome (leads V1 and V6).

During sinus rhythm the atrial impulse will be conducted to the ventricles by both the bundle of Kent and the normal AV node. Because the latter pathway conducts more slowly, initial ventricular activation is solely due to bundle of Kent conduction which results in ventricular pre-excitation and thus a shortened PR interval. Because the bundle of Kent is not connected to specialized conducting tissue, early ventricular activation will be relatively slow, leading to slurring of the ventricular complex and hence the delta wave. Once the atrial impulse has traversed the AV node, further ventricular activation will proceed normally. During sinus rhythm, therefore, the ventricular complex is a fusion between delta wave and normal QRS complex (*Fig.* 7.1).

Two main arrhythmias can occur in patients with the Wolff–Parkinson–White syndrome – atrial fibrillation and paroxysmal supraventricular tachycardia. The former, which is the less common of the two, is due to enhanced automaticity of an atrial ectopic focus, whereas the latter is caused by AV re-entry.

### Atrial Fibrillation

In patients without pre-excitation the ventricles are protected from the very rapid atrial activity during atrial fibrillation (350–600 impulses/min) by the AV node. In the Wolff–Parkinson–White syndrome the bundle of Kent provides an additional route of access to the ventricles and is often capable of very frequent conduction. As a result ventricular rates during atrial fibrillation tend to be faster than in patients without pre-excitation and in some patients can be dangerously fast.

Usually, most conducted impulses reach the ventricles via the bundle of Kent and therefore lead to delta waves. The minority of impulses that reach the ventricles via the AV node produce normal QRS complexes. The resultant ECG will, as in all cases of atrial fibrillation, show an irregularly irregular ventricular response. Some ventricular complexes will be normal, most will be delta waves (*Figs.* 7.4, 7.5).

A very rapid ventricular response to atrial fibrillation can be dangerous. First, heart failure or shock can result. Secondly, if the ventricles are stimulated at a very fast rate there is a risk of ventricular fibrillation. The risk is mainly confined to those patients where the minimum interval between delta waves during atrial fibrillation is less than 250 ms (*Fig.* 7.6).

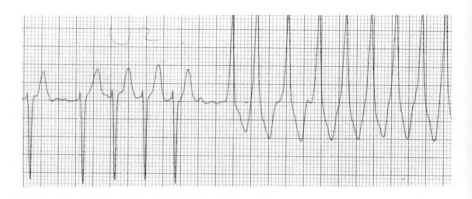

*Fig.* 7.4. Atrial fibrillation (lead V2). The first five complexes are conducted by the AV node and the last nine are conducted by the bundle of Kent and consist therefore of large delta waves.

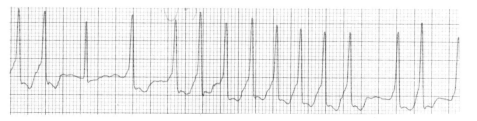

*Fig.* 7.5. Atrial fibrillation (lead V5). Only the third complex is a normally conducted beat, the other complexes are delta waves. There is the characteristic totally irregular ventricular response.

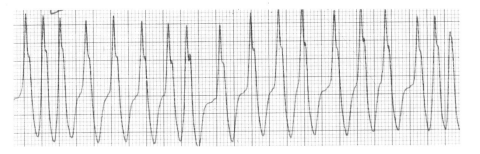

*Fig.* 7.6. Atrial fibrillation with a very rapid ventricular response (lead V1). The minimum interval between delta waves is 180 ms. The totally irregular response excludes a diagnosis of ventricular tachycardia.

## *Paroxysmal Supraventricular Tachycardia*

The AV junction and bundle of Kent differ in the time they take to recover after excitation. Usually, the AV junction recovers first. If an atrial ectopic beat arises during sinus rhythm, when the AV junction has recovered but the bundle of Kent is not yet capable of conduction, the resultant ventricular complex will clearly not have a delta wave and will be narrow. By the time the premature atrial impulse has traversed the AV junction and stimulated the ventricles, the bundle of Kent will have recovered and will be capable of conducting the impulse back to the atria. When the impulse reaches the atria the AV junction will again be capable of conduction and hence the impulse can repeatedly circulate between atria and ventricles. This circus movement is the mechanism causing paroxysmal supraventricular tachycardia in patients with the Wolff–Parkinson–White syndrome. Ventricular ectopic beats may, by a similar process, find one part of the circuit refractory to excitation and initiate a tachycardia.

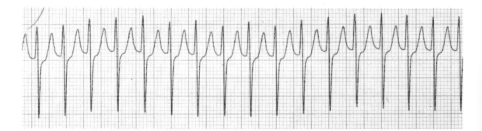

*Fig.* 7.7. Paroxysmal supraventricular tachycardia due to Wolff–Parkinson–White syndrome.

The ECG during tachycardia will show narrow ventricular complexes (unless phasic aberrant intraventricular conduction occurs) in rapid, regular succession (*Fig.* 7.7). Unlike atrial fibrillation, there will be no delta waves and, thus, there will be no clue from the appearance of the ventricular complexes during tachycardia that the patient has Wolff–Parkinson–White syndrome. However, the timing of atrial activity, if it can be identified, during tachycardia may give a clue as to its mechanism. When the tachycardia is due to two pathways within the AV node, i.e. 'dual AV nodal pathway' or 'intranodal' tachycardia (*see* Chapter 6), an inverted P wave immediately follows or is superimposed on the QRS complex. In contrast, in tachycardias due to the Wolff–Parkinson–White syndrome, the P wave occurs roughly halfway between QRS complexes (*Fig.* 7.8).

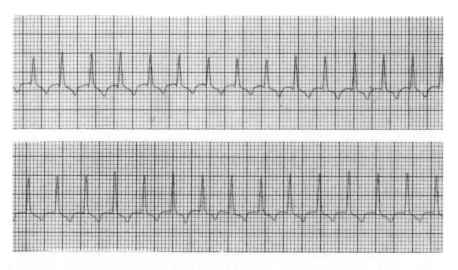

*Fig.* 7.8. Paroxysmal supraventricular tachycardia due to Wolff–Parkinson–White syndrome (leads II and AVF). Inverted P waves can be seen halfway between QRS complexes.

*Concealed Pre-excitation*

Many patients with paroxysmal supraventricular tachycardia who have no evidence of pre-excitation during sinus rhythm have been found to have a 'concealed' bundle of Kent when studied by intracardiac electrophysiological testing (*see* Chater 19).

The difference between concealed and ordinary bundles of Kent is that the former can only conduct in one direction. They can transmit impulses from ventricles to atria, the direction necessary to facilitate supraventricular tachycardia, but cannot conduct from atria to ventricles and thus there will be no delta wave or PR interval shortening.

Concealed pre-excitation should be suspected in a patient with a normal ECG during sinus rhythm when, during tachycardia, an inverted P wave is seen halfway between QRS complexes. If inverted in lead I, the bundle of Kent is likely to be left-sided (*Fig.* 7.9).

## Treatment

It is often asked, 'What is the treatment for Wolff–Parkinson–White syndrome?' There is no specific 'best' drug or other form of treatment for this syndrome.

*Paroxysmal Supraventricular Tachycardia*

Methods for the termination and prevention of paroxysmal supraventricular (i.e. AV re-entrant) tachycardia are discussed in Chapter 6. The methods are appropriate whether or not the patient has evidence of pre-excitation during sinus rhythm.

*Atrial Fibrillation*

During atrial fibrillation, most atrial impulses reach the ventricles via the accessory AV pathway. Thus, AV nodal-blocking drugs such as digoxin and verapamil, which are so useful in controlling atrial fibrillation in the absence of pre-excitation, are of little use in the Wolff–Parkinson–White syndrome. Indeed, both digoxin and verapamil can actually increase the frequency of conduction in the bundle of Kent and therefore lead to a faster ventricular rate. For this reason, these drugs should be avoided in those patients who are capable of a rapid ventricular response in case a dangerously fast ventricular rate develops. In patients in whom atrial fibrillation has never occurred, and thus a fast response has not been excluded, digoxin is best avoided.

The simplest method of terminating atrial fibrillation is cardioversion, but this is clearly not appropriate if the arrhythmia is frequently recurrent. If drugs are to be used, they must slow conduction in the bundle of Kent, e.g. intravenous disopyramide, sotalol, amiodarone or flecainide. These drugs will certainly slow the ventricular response to atrial

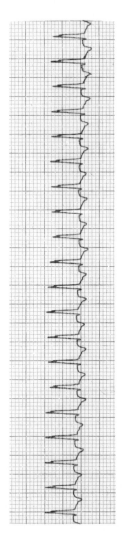

*Fig.* 7.9. Paroxysmal supraventricular tachycardia due to a concealed bundle of Kent (lead I). There is an inverted P wave superimposed on the T wave, halfway between QRS complexes.

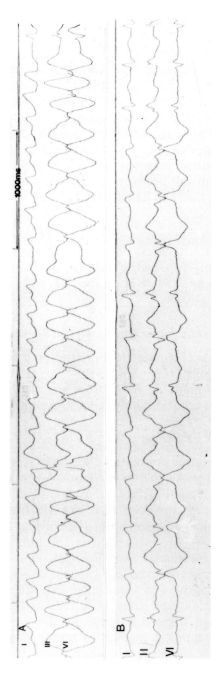

*Fig.* 7.10. Atrial fibrillation in a patient with type A Wolff—Parkinson—White syndrome before (A) and after (B) intravenous disopyramide. ECGs were recorded at 100 mm/s. The minimum interval between delta waves has increased from 180 ms to 400 ms.

fibrillation (the latter two are the most potent) and will often effect a return to sinus rhythm.

For prevention of atrial fibrillation oral quinidine, disopyramide, sotalol or flecainide can be used. In patients with a dangerously fast ventricular response to atrial fibrillation it may be worth initiating atrial fibrillation by rapid atrial pacing once the patient is established on an anti-arrhythmic drug to ensure that the drug will slow the ventricular response to atrial fibrillation.

Surgical division of the bundle of Kent may be necessary when drugs are ineffective or cannot be tolerated, especially if the ventricular response is very fast.

## LOWN–GANONG–LEVINE SYNDROME

The characteristics of the syndrome are a short PR interval, a normal QRS complex and a tendency to paroxysmal tachycardia.

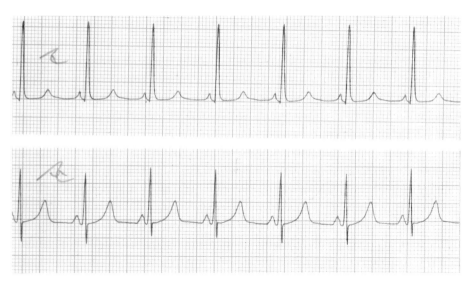

*Fig.* 7.11.   Lown–Ganong–Levine syndrome (leads I and II). The·PR interval is short but the QRS complex is normal.

In this pre-excitation syndrome there is an additional AV connection between atrial myocardium and the bundle of His, which therefore bypasses the AV node. Thus, an atrial impulse will reach the ventricles without the normal delay and lead to a very short PR interval. Because the tract is connected to the Bundle of His, ventricular activation will be normal and, therefore, there will not be a delta wave (*Fig.* 7.11).

Patients with this syndrome are prone to episodes of paroxysmal supraventricular tachycardia which should be treated in the normal way.

Intracardiac electrophysiological studies have revealed that some patients with the Lown—Ganong—Levine syndrome also have a bundle of Kent.

Not all patients with a short PR interval have an AV nodal bypass tract or are prone to paroxysmal tachycardia.

## Main Points

1. The Wolff–Parkinson–White syndrome is characterized by a short PR interval, a widened QRS complex due to presence of a delta wave and a tendency to paroxysmal tachycardia. It is caused by an accessory AV pathway (bundle of Kent), which connects atrial and ventricular myocardium, bypassing the AV junction.

2. Two main arrhythmias can occur: paroxysmal supraventricular tachycardia (AV re-entrant tachycardia) and atrial fibrillation.

3. During paroxysmal supraventricular tachycardia, there will be no delta waves and thus no evidence from the ventricular complex that there is pre-excitation. The management of the arrhythmia is the same whether or not there is pre-excitation.

4. During atrial fibrillation, most ventricular complexes are broad due to the presence of large delta waves. The ventricular rate is often very fast and there is a risk of ventricular fibrillation being initiated when the minimum interval between delta waves during atrial fibrillation is less than 250 ms. If the hallmark of atrial fibrillation (i.e. a totally irregular rhythm) is ignored, ventricular tachycardia may be mistakenly diagnosed.

5. Since most atrial impulses are conducted to the ventricles via the accessory AV pathway during atrial fibrillation, AV nodal-blocking drugs are not helpful. Cardioversion is the simplest method for termination of atrial fibrillation. If drugs are to be used, they must be ones which impair conduction in the accessory pathway (e.g. disopyramide, sotalol, flecainide and amiodarone).

6. The Lown–Ganong–Levine syndrome is characterized by a short PR interval, normal QRS complex and tendency to paroxysmal tachycardia. It is caused by an accessory AV connection between atrial myocardium and the bundle of His. (Paroxysmal supraventricular tachycardia should be treated in the normal way.) Not all patients with a short PR interval have this syndrome.

Chapter *8*

# Tachycardias with Broad Ventricular Complexes

Tachycardias of supraventricular origin are sometimes associated with bundle branch block and hence broad ventricular complexes. They may thus mimic ventricular tachycardia. Now that it is widely appreciated that this can occur, the tendency is to misinterpret ventricular tachycardia as supraventricular, rather than the reverse.

Tachycardias with broad ventricular complexes can be due to:

Ventricular tachycardia.

Supraventricular tachycardia when bundle branch block has already been present during sinus rhythm.

Supraventricular tachycardia with phasic aberrant intraventricular conduction (i.e. rate-related bundle branch block).

## USELESS GUIDELINES

It is often said that whereas ventricular tachycardia leads to major haemo-dynamic disturbance, supraventricular tachycardia does not. This is incorrect. Sometimes ventricular tachycardia, even due to recent myocardial infarction, causes few or even no symptoms, whereas supraventricular tachycardia, particularly if very fast or in the presence of underlying heart disease, can sometimes cause shock or heart failure.

Another widely quoted rule is that whereas supraventricular tachy-cardia is regular, ventricular tachycardia is slightly irregular. This rule is unreliable. Ventricular tachycardia is usually regular unless there are capture beats.

## USEFUL GUIDELINES

### Ventricular Tachycardia and Coronary Artery or Myocardial Disease

Ventricular tachycardia is a common arrhythmia in patients with coronary artery or myocardial disease. On the other hand, paroxysmal (AV re-entrant) supraventricular tachycardia virtually never occurs unless the patient was already prone to it: coronary or myocardial disease will not create the additional electrical connection between atria and ventricles that is necessary to facilitate this arrhythmia.

Atrial fibrillation and flutter (*Figs.* 8.1, 8.2) are two arrhythmias of

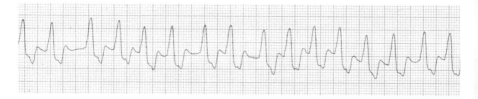

*Fig.* 8.1. Atrial fibrillation with left bundle branch block (lead V6). The ventricular rhythm is totally irregular.

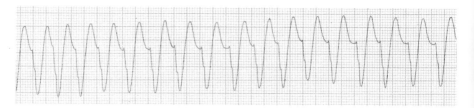

*Fig.* 8.2. Another example of atrial fibrillation with left bundle branch block (lead V3). Though the ventricular rate is more rapid, the rhythm is totally irregular, thus excluding ventricular tachycardia.

supraventricular origin which may be caused by coronary or myocardial disease and may sometimes be associated with broad ventricular complexes. However, these arrhythmias have characteristic features whose recognition should prevent confusion with ventricular tachycardia (*see* Chapter 6). Thus in a patient with coronary artery or myocardial disease, a regular tachycardia with broad ventricular complexes is likely to be ventricular in origin, even if there is little haemodynamic disturbance.

## Ectopic Beats

If the configuration of the ventricular complex during tachycardia is similar to that of an ectopic beat recorded during normal rhythm, a common origin is probable. It is relatively easy to ascertain the origin of single ectopic beats, especially if a full ECG is available (*Fig.* 8.3). ·

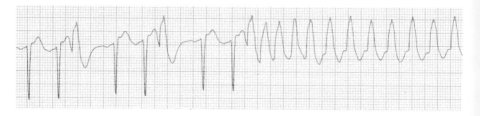

*Fig.* 8.3. The third ventricular ectopic beat initiates ventricular tachycardia.

## Independent Atrial Activity

If independent atrial activity (*see* Chapter 5) can be identified directly (*Fig.* 8.4) or indirectly (*Fig.* 8.5) then supraventricular tachycardia is excluded. (Strictly speaking, independent atrial activity can occur in some

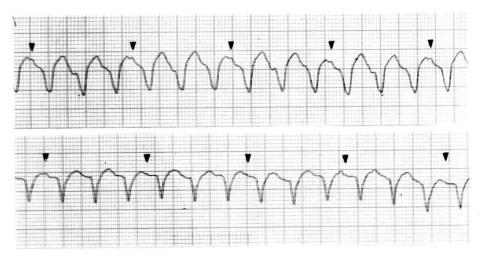

*Fig.* 8.4. Independent atrial activity during ventricular tachycardia (leads AVF and V1). Dissociated atrial activity at intervals of 1·04 s can be identified (arrowheads).

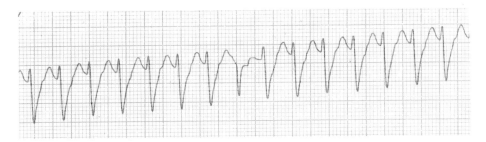

*Fig.* 8.5. Ventricular tachycardia (lead II). The eighth complex is a capture beat.

cases of junctional tachycardia when there is no retrograde conduction to the atria. For practical purposes, however, such a tachycardia is ventricular, since AV nodal-blocking drugs will not be helpful.)

As discussed in Chapter 5, scrutiny of several ECG leads may be necessary to identify evidence of atrial activity (*Fig.* 8.6).

In some patients an atrial electrocardiogram, recorded simultaneously with a surface ECG, is necessary to demonstrate independent atrial activity (*Fig.* 8.7). An atrial electrogram can be obtained by passing a transvenous electrode to the right atrium or by using an oesophageal electrode positioned behind the left atrium. An electrically isolated or battery powered ECG recorder should be used.

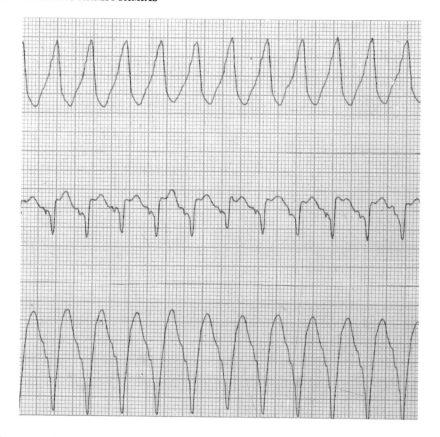

*Fig.* 8.6. Advantage of simultaneous recording of ECG leads (I, II and III). Lead II suggests that there may be a P wave before each QRS complex and thus that the tachycardia is supraventricular in origin rather than ventricular. However, comparison with other leads indicates that the 'P' wave is in fact the initial vector of the ventricular complex.

## Carotid Sinus Massage

Carotid sinus massage can slow AV node conduction and may thus terminate paroxysmal supraventricular tachycardia. If a reduction in ventricular rate occurs during massage but sinus rhythm does not return, it is likely that the patient has atrial flutter or fibrillation; with a higher degree of AV block, flutter and fibrillation waves are more easily identifiable.

Carotid sinus massage is not always effective in paroxysmal supraventricular tachycardia and its failure cannot be taken as evidence for ventricular tachycardia.

## Configuration of Ventricular Complex

Supraventricular tachycardia may cause bundle branch block, i.e. phasic aberrant intraventricular conduction (*Fig.* 8.8). It is usually the right

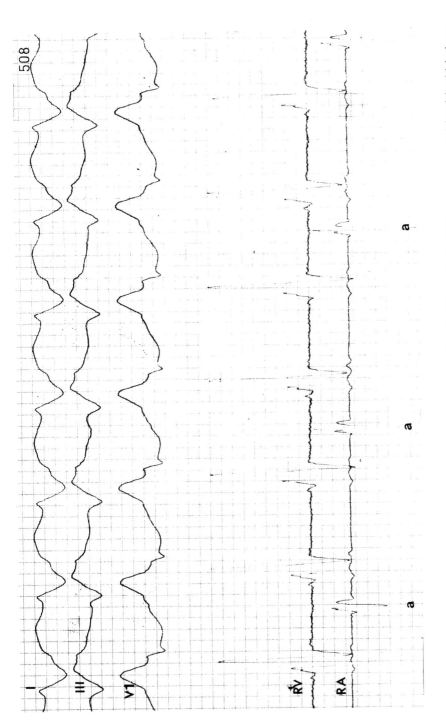

*Fig. 8.7.* Leads I, III and V1 recorded at 100 mm/s with right atrial (RA) and right ventricular (RV) electrograms. Atrial activity (a) is slower than and independent of ventricular activity, indicating ventricular tachycardia.

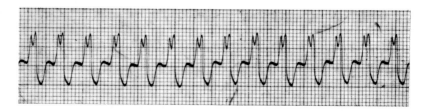

*Fig.* 8.8. Supraventricular tachycardia with left bundle branch block aberration in a case of Wolff–Parkinson–White syndrome (lead V5).

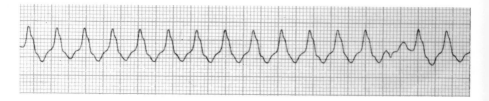

*Fig.* 8.9. Ventricular tachycardia (lead V1). The appearance of the complexes is of right bundle branch block type.

bundle which is blocked. Ventricular tachycardia originating from the left ventricle can also result in ventricular complexes with right bundle branch block appearance but there are differences. In ventricular tachycardia, the complex in lead V1 is usually biphasic and often has a small Q wave, whereas in aberrant conduction the complex is triphasic and always has an initial positive wave (*Fig.* 8.9).

### Retrograde Concealed Conduction

As discussed in Chapter 3, partial penetration of the AV node by a ventricular ectopic impulse may lead to prolongation of the PR interval during the subsequent sinus beat. Prolongation of the PR interval in the first sinus beat after a tachycardia indicates a ventricular origin.

## Main Points

1. Though tachycardias of supraventricular origin can be associated with bundle branch block and hence broad QRS complexes, most broad complex tachycardias are ventricular in origin.

2. Neither the regularity of an arrhythmia nor haemodynamic status are useful in distinguishing supraventricular from ventricular tachycardia.

3. A regular tachycardia with broad ventricular complexes in association with coronary artery or myocardial disease is almost certainly of ventricular origin.

**4.** Direct evidence of independent atrial activity or the presence of capture or fusion beats indicates ventricular tachycardia.

**5.** When supraventricular tachycardia is associated with aberrant intra-ventricular conduction, the morphology of the ventricular complexes is usually that of classic left or right bundle branch block.

# Chapter 9

# Atrioventricular Block

The most common cause of atrioventricular (AV) block is idiopathic fibrosis of the AV junction or bundle branches. Other causes include:

Myocardial infarction
Digoxin toxicity
Aortic valve disease
Congenital isolated lesion
Congenital heart disease, e.g. corrected transposition
Cardiac surgery
Infiltration, e.g. tumour, sarcoidosis, syphilis, endocarditis
Inflammation, e.g. ankylosing spondylitis, Reiter's syndrome, rheumatoid arthritis, scleroderma
Rheumatic fever
Dystrophia myotonica
Diphtheria

AV block is classified as first, second or third degree depending on whether conduction of atrial impulses to the ventricles is delayed, intermittently blocked or completely blocked.

## FIRST DEGREE AV BLOCK

Conduction of the atrial impulse to the ventricles is delayed, resulting in prolongation of the PR interval (*Figs.* 9.1–9.3). The PR interval is measured from the onset of the P wave to the onset of the ventricular complex – whether this be a Q or an R wave – and is prolonged if it is greater than 0·21 s.

Usually conduction is delayed in the AV node, but rarely delay occurs within the atria or bundle of His.

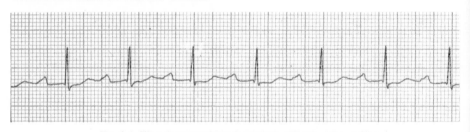

*Fig.* 9.1. First degree AV block (lead II). PR interval = 0·28 s.

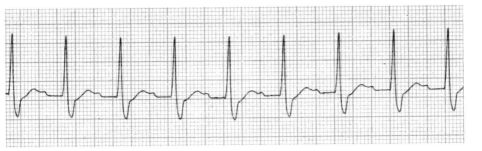

*Fig.* 9.2. First degree AV block and sinus tachycardia (lead I). PR interval = 0·24 s.

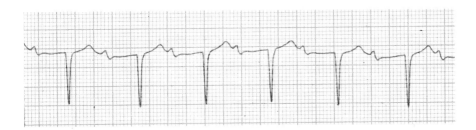

*Fig.* 9.3. First degree AV block (lead V1). The P wave is superimposed on the terminal portion of the preceding T wave. PR interval = 0·38 s.

First degree AV block does not cause symptoms but may progress to higher degrees of block. In young persons it may be a benign phenomenon due to high vagal tone.

## SECOND DEGREE AV BLOCK

In second degree AV block there is intermittent failure of conduction of atrial impulses to the ventricles, leading to dropped beats, i.e. P waves not followed by QRS complexes. Second degree block is subdivided into Mobitz type I (Wenkebach) and Mobitz type II block.

### Mobitz Type I or Wenkebach AV Block

In this form of second degree block AV conduction becomes progressively more delayed with each atrial impulse until there is complete block and an atrial impulse fails to be conducted to the ventricles. After the dropped beat, AV conduction recovers and the sequence starts again (*Figs.* 9.4, 9.5).

A V Wenkebach block is due to impaired conduction in the AV node. Like first AV block, it can be benign (particularly when observed during sleep), being due to high vagal tone.

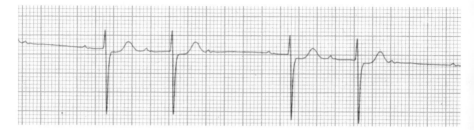

*Fig.* 9.4. AV Wenkebach block. Unlike many textbooks examples, but as often occurs in practice, the trace does not start with the shortest PR interval.

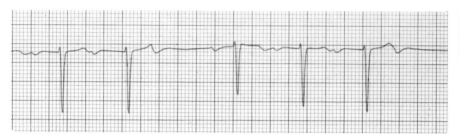

*Fig.* 9.5. AV Wenkebach block. The non-conducted P wave is superimposed on the preceding T wave.

The increments in AV-nodal conduction delay are usually greatest at the start of the Wenkebach sequence. This leads to the somewhat paradoxical finding that, as the sequence approaches the dropped beat, the QRS complexes actually become closer together.

### Mobitz Type II AV Block

In Mobitz type II block there is intermittent failure of conduction of atrial impulses to the ventricles without antecedent progressive lengthening of the PR interval, and thus the PR interval of conducted beats is constant (*Fig.* 9.6).

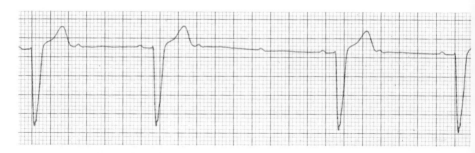

*Fig.* 9.6. Mobitz type II AV block. In this example the ratio between conducted and non-conducted atrial impulses varies.

In contrast to first degree and Wenkebach AV block, Mobitz type II block is usually due to impaired conduction in the bundle of His or bundle branches (i.e. infranodal). Thus, because there is bundle branch disease, the QRS complexes are usually broad. Block below the AV node is more likely to be associated with Stokes—Adams attacks, slow ventricular rates and sudden death.

The ratio of conducted to non-conducted atrial impulses varies. Commonly 2 : 1 AV conduction occurs (*Fig.* 9.7). A similar pattern may be caused by an extreme form of Wenkebach block so that it is difficult to make prognostic inferences from 2 : 1 AV block (*Fig.* 9.8).

Usually, during Mobitz type II block, the atrial rate is regular. Sometimes, however, the P–P interval encompassing a ventricular complex is shorter than a P–P interval which does not. This is known as ventriculophasic sinus arrhythmia.

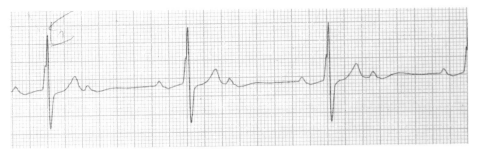

*Fig.* 9.7. Mobitz type II AV block with 2 : 1 AV conduction.

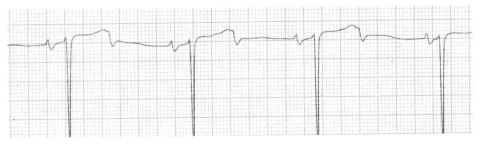

*Fig.* 9.8. 2 : 1 AV block with narrow QRS complexes (lead V1). The non-conducted atrial beats are superimposed on preceding T waves.

## THIRD DEGREE AV BLOCK

Third degree or complete AV block occurs when there is total interruption of the transmission of atrial impulses to the ventricles. Third degree block may be due to interrupted conduction at either AV nodal or infranodal level. When the block is within the AV node, subsidiary pacemakers arise within the bundle of His and, unless there is additional bundle branch block, will lead to narrow QRS complexes (*Fig.* 9.9). Often, pacemakers within the bundle of His discharge reliably at a fairly rapid rate.

In contrast, in infranodal block subsidiary pacemakers usually arise in the left or right bundle branches. These pacemakers will produce broad QRS complexes and slower ventricular rates (*Figs.* 9.10, 9.13). Pacemaker activity is less reliable and thus Stokes—Adams attacks are more likely.

Complete AV block can complicate atrial fibrillation and flutter (*Figs.* 9.11, 9.12).

## Supernormal Conduction

Occasionally, even during third degree AV block, atrial impulses may be conducted to the ventricles. There is a short period immediately after recovery from excitation when AV conduction may transiently improve. This period usually coincides with inscription of the latter portion of the T wave (*Fig.* 9.13). As a result, atrial impulses falling on this part of the T wave will be followed by a premature QRS complex.

## AV DISSOCIATION

During third degree AV block, atrial activity is faster than and dissociated from ventricular activity. Dissociation between atrial and ventricular activity also occurs when, often during sinus bradycardia, an escape rhythm faster than the sinus rate arises in the AV junction or ventricles (*Fig.* 9.14). The term 'AV dissociation' should be reserved for this latter situation, in which the ventricular rate is *greater* than the atrial rate. If AV dissociation is not distinguished from complete AV block, inappropriate action can result.  For example, AV dissociation often occurs in acute myocardial infarction and, if not recognized as such, a pacemaker may be unnecessarily inserted.

During AV dissociation, the timing of some P waves may be such that they can be transmitted by the AV junction and capture the ventricles before the next discharge from the escape junctional or ventricular focus and therefore lead to premature ventricular activation. This is known as 'AV dissociation with capture beats'.

## BILATERAL BUNDLE BRANCH DISEASE

Infranodal AV block may be due to a lesion in the bundle of His but is more often caused by disease in both left and right bundle branches.

Although the anatomical situation may be more complex, functionally the bundle of His can be considered to divide into three: the right bundle branch and the anterior and posterior fascicles of the left bundle branch (*see* Chapter 4).

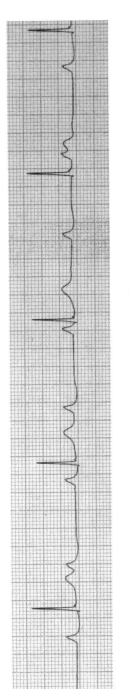

*Fig.* 9.9. Complete AV block with narrow QRS complexes.

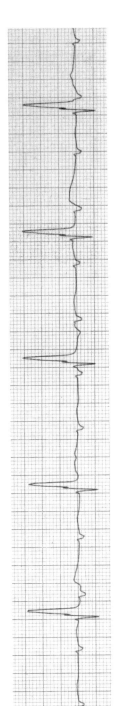

*Fig.* 9.10. Complete AV block with broad QRS complexes.

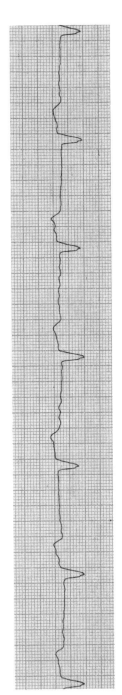

*Fig.* 9.11. Complete AV block with atrial fibrillation.

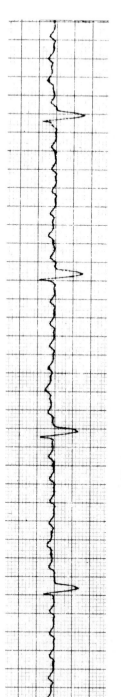

*Fig.* 9.12. Complete AV block with atrial flutter.

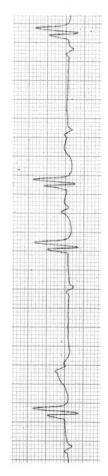

*Fig.* 9.13. Complete AV block. There is supernormal conduction of the atrial impulse that falls on the T wave of the second ventricular complex (lead V1).

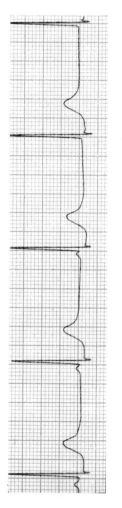

*Fig.* 9.14. AV dissociation. Atrial and ventricular rates are 49 and 51/min, respectively. The fourth and fifth P waves are concealed by superimposed QRS complexes.

If conduction is blocked in only two of the three fascicles (bifascicular block), the functioning fascicle will conduct atrial impulses to the ventricles and maintain sinus rhythm. Block in the third fascicle will lead to complete AV block.

## Bifascicular Block

The most common pattern of bifascicular block is right bundle branch plus left anterior fascicular block (*Fig.* 9.15). The posterior fascicle of the left bundle branch is a stouter structure and has a better blood supply than the anterior fascicle and is therefore less vulnerable. As a result, right bundle branch plus left posterior fascicular block is a less frequent occurrence (*Fig.* 9.16).

Block in both anterior and posterior fascicles of the left bundle branch causes complete left bundle branch block. The combination of left bundle branch block and left axis deviation may indicate more severe disease of conduction tissues than left bundle branch block with a normal frontal axis (*Fig.* 9.17).

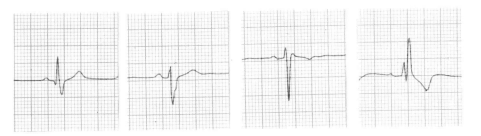

*Fig.* 9.15. Left anterior fascicular and right bundle branch block (leads I, II, III and V1).

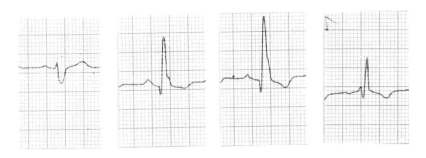

*Fig.* 9.16. Left posterior fascicular and right bundle branch block (leads I, II, III and V1).

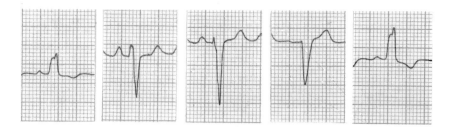

*Fig.* 9.17. Left axis deviation and left bundle branch block (leads I, II, III, V1 and V6).

PR interval prolongation is usually due to impaired AV node conduction, but in the context of bifascicular block it is more likely to reflect abnormal conduction in the functioning fascicle.

## Trifascicular Block

Interrupted conduction in all three fascicles results in complete AV block. In many patients one of the three fascicles is capable of intermittent conduction so that, for part of the time, there will be sinus rhythm with evidence of bifascicular block.

The risk of bifascicular block progressing to trifascicular block is fairly low. In patients with right bundle and left anterior fascicular block, this is in the order of a few per cent per year. The risk is increased when there is right bundle and left posterior fascicular block and when there is alternating complete right and left bundle branch block. There is little evidence to suggest that prophylactic implantation of a permanent pacemaker in asymptomatic patients with bifascicular block improves prognosis. The major determinants of prognosis are the states of the myocardium and coronary arteries.

## CLINICAL FEATURES OF AV BLOCK

First degree and Mobitz type I second degree AV block do not cause symptoms but may progress to higher grades of block.

In Mobitz type II and complete AV block, a low ventricular rate may cause tiredness, dyspnoea and heart failure. In some patients the ventricular pacemaker may at times discharge very slowly or actually stop, leading to syncope or, if ventricular activity does not quickly return, sudden death. Ventricular fibrillation and tachycardia arise in some patients as a consequence of the low ventricular rate and may also lead to syncope or sudden death.

### Stokes—Adams Attacks

Syncope due to transient asystole or ventricular fibrillation – a Stokes—Adams attack – has characteristic features. These features are of great diagnostic importance because, on the one hand, abnormalities of AV conduction (and sinus node function) may be intermittent, routine electrocardiography being normal, and on the other hand, in patients with evidence of disease of the specialized conducting tissues, syncope may be due to unrelated causes such as epilepsy.

In a Stokes—Adams attack, loss of consciousness is abrupt. There is virtually no warning, though the patient will sometimes feel that he is going to faint, just before he loses consciousness. The patient collapses, lying motionless, pale and pulseless. He looks as though he is dead. In a prolonged attack twitching may develop and progress to a fit. Usually, within a minute or two, consciousness returns, and as cardiac action resumes there is a vivid flush to the skin. Incontinence does occur occasionally but is not a regular feature as it is in epilepsy. Unlike epilepsy, recovery is quick and confusion and headache after the attack are unusual.

In some patients the rhythm disturbance does not last long enough to cause syncope but the patient feels as though he is going to faint (near-syncope) and then recovers. He may complain of 'dizziness' but will not experience true vertigo.

### Congenital Heart Block

This is a relatively benign disorder. AV conduction is interrupted at AV nodal level. Consequently, the subsidiary ventricular pacemaker is situated in the proximal part of the bundle of His (producing narrow QRS complexes) and discharges reliably at a relatively fast rate (40—80/min) which may accelerate on exercise. In most cases there are no symptoms and exercise tolerance is good.

However, syncope and sudden death do occur in a minority of patients and may be more common in those with prolonged QTc interval and in those with frequent ventricular extrasystoles.

### Acquired Heart Block

Heart block complicating myocardial infarction is discussed in Chapter 11.

As discussed above, the commonest cause of heart block is idiopathic fibrosis of the AV junction or bundle branches. This mainly affects the elderly but — as with the other causes of AV block — can affect the young and middle aged as well.

The bradycardia associated with Mobitz type II and third degree AV block may reduce cardiac output and lead to symptoms such as shortness of breath, tiredness and heart failure. Stokes—Adams attacks will sooner or later occur in about two-thirds of patients with these higher grades of AV block.

The prognosis of patients with AV block depends on three main factors. First, the presence of associated cardiac disease (for example, the prognosis is poor in those patients with coronary artery disease). Secondly, the site of AV block (patients with infranodal AV block have a poorer prognosis than those with nodal block). Thirdly, the prognosis is worse in patients with syncope.

### Treatment

Artificial cardiac pacing has greatly improved the symptoms and prognosis. The indications are discussed in Chapters 15 and 16.

## Main Points

1. AV block is classified as first, second or third degree depending on whether conduction of atrial impulses to the ventricles is delayed, intermittently blocked or completely blocked.

2. Second degree AV block is subdivided into Mobitz I (Wenkebach) and Mobitz II types. In the former, there is progressive lengthening of the PR interval prior to non-conduction of an atrial impulse, whereas the PR interval of conducted atrial impulses is constant in Mobitz II.

3. During AV dissociation (in contrast to complete AV block), the atrial rate is slower than the ventricular rate.

4. First degree block, Wenkebach block and third degree block with narrow QRS complexes are due to disease within the AV node, whereas Mobitz II and complete block with broad QRS complexes are likely to be due to infranodal block.

5. Bifascicular block may deteriorate intermittently or permanently to complete (trifascicular) AV block.

6. Stokes–Adams attacks are characterized by abrupt loss of consciousness which lasts for a few minutes only, following which recovery is usually rapid. Patients with conduction tissue disease often experience 'near-syncope' as well as episodes of complete loss of consciousness.

# Chapter 10

# Sick Sinus Syndrome

The sick sinus syndrome, also referred to as sino-atrial disease, is caused by impairment of either sinus node activity or of conduction of impulses from the sinus node to the atria. The result is sinus bradycardia, sino-atrial block or sinus arrest.

In some patients tachycardias of supraventricular origin may also occur. The term 'bradycardia–tachycardia' (often abbreviated to 'brady–tachy') syndrome is applied to these patients.

Sick sinus syndrome is a common cause of syncope, dizzy attacks and palpitation. Though found most frequently in the elderly, it can occur at any age.

## CAUSES

In most cases the cause is idiopathic fibrosis of the sinus node. Sick sinus syndrome can be due to acute myocardial infarction, chronic ischaemic heart disease, cardiomyopathy, myocarditis, digoxin or quinidine toxicity, or cardiac surgery, especially atrial septal defect repair. Sometimes, anti-arrhythmic drugs may precipitate an otherwise latent disorder.

## ECG CHARACTERISTICS

Any one of the following abnormal rhythms can occur. They are often intermittent, normal sinus rhythm being present for most of the time.

### Sinus Bradycardia

Sinus bradycardia is a common finding in the sick sinus syndrome. The rate may fall as low as 30 beats/min.

### Sinus Arrest

Sinus arrest is due to failure of the sinus node to activate the atria because of cessation of sinus node activity. The result is absence of normal P waves (*Figs.* 10.1, 10.2).

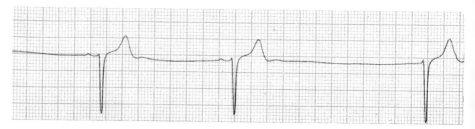

*Fig.* 10.1. Sinus bradycardia and then sinus arrest leading to a junctional escape beat.

Physiological studies have shown that in the absence of sinus node activity, subsidiary pacemakers in the atria, AV junction or ventricles should give rise to an escape rhythm. In the sick sinus syndrome, however, the subsidiary pacemakers are often far from reliable and sinus arrest may therefore lead to cardiac standstill. Thus, although sinus arrest is attributed to disordered sinus node function, where asystole occurs, there is also abnormal function of the more distal specialized conducting system (*Fig.* 10.2).

It should be noted that sinus bradycardia and sinoatrial block during sleep are physiological and should not be taken as evidence for the sick sinus syndrome. Furthermore, pauses in sinus node activity of up to 2.0 s due to high vagal tone may be found in fit, young people.

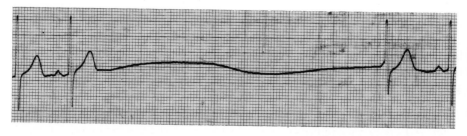

*Fig.* 10.2. Sinus arrest leading to a prolonged period of ventricular standstill, eventually terminated by a junctional escape beat.

## Sino-atrial Block

Sino-atrial block occurs when sinus node impulses fail to traverse the junction between the node and surrounding atrial myocardium. Like atrioventricular block, sino-atrial block can be classified into first, second or third degree. However, only second degree sino-atrial block can be confidently diagnosed from the ECG. Third degree or complete sino-atrial block is indistinguishable from sinus arrest.

In second degree sino-atrial block, there are intermittently dropped P waves, resulting in intervals between P waves which are multiples of (often twice) the cycle length during sinus rhythm (*Fig.* 10.3).

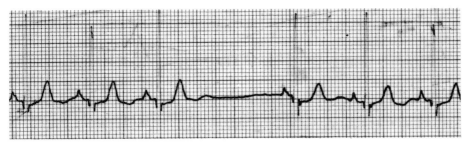

*Fig.* 10.3.  Second degree sino-atrial block. Both the P wave and QRS complex are dropped for one cycle.

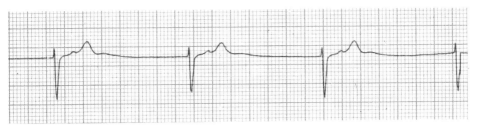

*Fig.* 10.4.  Junctional escape rhythm secondary to sinus arrest. The junctional focus activates the atria retrogradely leading to P waves superimposed on the ST segments.

### Escape Beats and Rhythms

When sinus bradycardia or arrest occurs, subsidiary pacemakers may give rise to an escape beat or rhythm (*Fig.* 10.1, 10.2, 10.4). Presence of a junctional or idioventricular rhythm suggests abnormal sinus node function.

### Atrial Ectopic Beats

These are often found in the sick sinus syndrome (*Fig.* 10.5). Characteristically they are followed by long pauses because sinus node automaticity is depressed by the ectopic beat (*Fig.* 10.6).

## BRADYCARDIA–TACHYCARDIA  SYNDROME

Several tachycardias of supraventricular origin may occur in patients with the sick sinus syndrome. Paroxysmal atrial fibrillation and flutter are the most common (*Fig.* 10.5). Atrial and junctional tachycardia also occur (*Fig.* 10.7). However, paroxysmal supraventricular (i.e. AV nodal re-entrant) tachycardia (*see* Chapter 6) is not associated with this syndrome.

Sinus node automaticity is often depressed by these tachycardias so that termination of the tachycardia is followed by a period of sinus bradycardia or arrest. Conversely, tachycardias often arise as an escape rhythm following bradycardia. Thus, tachycardia often alternates with bradycardia.

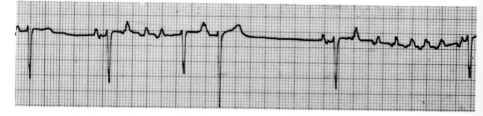

*Fig.* 10.5 Atrial ectopic beats after the second, third and fifth QRS complexes. On two occasions brief episodes of atrial flutter are initiated.

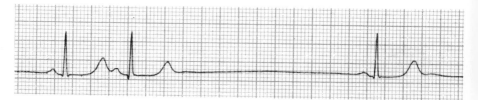

*Fig.* 10.6.   Atrial ectopic beat leads to depression of sinus node automaticity.

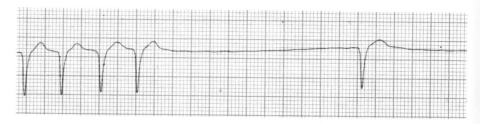

*Fig.* 10.7.   Termination of junctional tachycardia followed by sinus arrest.

## AV JUNCTION DISEASE

Abnormal AV conduction is not infrequently found in patients with sick sinus syndrome (*Fig.* 10.8). In patients with sick sinus syndrome who develop atrial fibrillation there is often a slow ventricular response in the absence of digoxin or other AV nodal-blocking drugs suggesting coexistent impaired AV nodal function (*Fig.* 10.9).

## CLINICAL FEATURES

Sinus arrest without an adequate escape rhythm may cause syncope or dizzy attacks, depending on its duration. Tachycardias often produce palpitation, and resultant sinus node depression may lead to syncope or near-syncope after palpitation.

The frequency of rhythm disturbance is very variable. Some patients will experience symptoms many times per day whereas in others symptoms may be separated by intervals of several months.

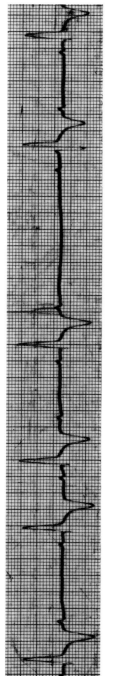

*Fig.* 10.8. Intermittent Mobitz type II AV block and periods of sinus arrest.

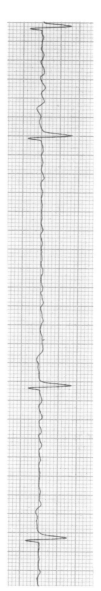

*Fig.* 10.9.    Atrial fibrillation with slow ventricular response in a patient who also had periods of sinus bradycardia and arrest.

In the absence of mitral valve disease, atrial tachyarrhythmias very rarely cause systemic embolism. The bradycardia–tachycardia syndrome is an exception to this rule. Incidences of up to 15 per cent have been reported.

## DIAGNOSIS

Sick sinus syndrome should be suspected when there are symptoms of syncope, near-syncope or palpitation in the presence of sinus bradycardia or an escape rhythm. Prolonged sinus arrest or sino-atrial block confirms the diagnosis.

Sometimes diagnostic information can be obtained from the standard ECG but often 24-hour ambulatory ECG recordings will be necessary.

Occasionally, when symptoms and rhythm disturbances are infrequent, intracardiac electrophysiological testing may be helpful (*see* Chapter 19).

## TREATMENT

### Sinus Bradycardia or Arrest

With the exception of sinus node dysfunction in acute myocardial infarction, where atropine may be helpful, drugs are ineffective in preventing sinus bradycardia or arrest and may precipitate tachyarrhythmias. Cardiac pacing is necessary to control symptoms.

For two reasons atrial pacing is preferable to ventricular pacing. First, atrial pacing maintains the normal sequence of cardiac chamber activation. With ventricular pacing the loss of atrial contribution to ventricular filling may result in a reduction of cardiac output of up to 30 per cent (*see* Chapter 16). The second advantage to atrial pacing is that regular atrial systole reduces the risk of systemic emboli. In patients with both sinus node and AV junction disease, A–V sequential pacing can be carried out (*see* Chapter 16).

### Bradycardia–Tachycardia Syndrome

Anti-arrhythmic drugs, especially beta-blockers and disopyramide, often worsen sinus node function and thus increase the risk of syncope. It is usually necessary to implant a pacemaker if anti-arrhythmic drugs are required to control tachycardias, particularly if sino-atrial block or arrest has occurred.

Tachycardias often arise as an escape rhythm during bradycardia. Atrial pacing may prevent initiation of tachyarrhythmias by ensuring regular atrial activity.

Cardioversion may cause asystole and should be preceded by insertion of a temporary pacemaker.

**Systemic Embolism**

Because of the risk of systemic embolism, some would recommend long term anticoagulation for patients in whom atrial tachyarrhythmias cannot be prevented. Anticoagulants are certainly indicated when there is a history of embolism.

## CAROTID SINUS SYNDROME

This term refers to a group of patients who suffer from near-syncope or syncope without electrocardiographic evidence of sinus node or AV junctional disease in whom unilateral carotid sinus massage (for 5 s) causes sinus arrest or complete AV block for 3 s or more. In some of these patients, baroreceptor stimulation also causes marked hypotension.

Furthermore, it should be noted that some subjects, particularly among the elderly, who are entirely asymptomatic, may develop a marked bradycardia on carotid massage. In symptomatic patients, atrial or AV sequential pacing is required.

## Main Points

1. The sick sinus syndrome is due to impaired sinus node function and/ or sino-atrial conduction and may cause sinus bradycardia, sino-atrial block or sinus arrest.

2. A substantial pause in sinus node activity without an adequate junctional or ventricular escape rhythm will cause near-syncope or syncope.

3. The bradycardia–tachycardia syndrome consists of the occurrence of both sinus node dysfunction and episodes of atrial fibrillation, flutter or tachycardia. Often, bradycardia will alternate with tachycardia. AV re-entrant tachycardia does not occur as part of this syndrome.

4. Artificial pacing is required for symptoms due to the sick sinus syndrome and to prevent profound bradycardia if anti-arrhythmic drugs are to be prescribed for the bradycardia–tachycardia syndrome.

# Chapter 11

# Arrhythmias in Myocardial Infarction

Myocardial infarction can cause a wide variety of arrhythmias. Some necessitate immediate treatment whereas no treatment is required for others. Some arrhythmias have no prognostic significance, whereas others are usually associated with extensive myocardial damage and imply a poor long-term prognosis.

## VENTRICULAR FIBRILLATION

Ventricular fibrillation is the rapid, totally incoordinate contraction of ventricular myocardial fibres. This is reflected in the ECG by irregular, chaotic electrical activity (*Fig.* 11.1). Ventricular fibrillation causes circulatory arrest and unconsciousness develops within a few seconds. Ventricular fibrillation is usually, but not always, initiated by an 'R on T' ventricular ectopic beat (*Fig.* 11.2).

Ninety per cent of deaths caused by myocardial infarction are due to ventricular fibrillation. The incidence of fibrillation is highest in the first hour after the onset of chest pain and diminishes progressively thereafter. Forty per cent of deaths occur within the first hour. Thus, many patients who are potentially treatable die before they can be admitted to hospital.

In those patients who reach hospital, however, ventricular fibrillation and other arrhythmias are sufficiently common to necessitate continuous ECG monitoring for 24–48 h in an area where facilities for resuscitation are immediately available, i.e. a coronary care unit.

Between 3 and 10 per cent of patients with acute myocardial infarction develop ventricular fibrillation while in a coronary case unit. The main determinant of incidence of ventricular fibrillation in a coronary care unit is the delay before admission: the shorter the delay, the greater the incidence of ventricular fibrillation.

When ventricular fibrillation develops in a heart that was functioning satisfactorily during normal rhythm it is termed 'primary' fibrillation, whereas if it occurs in the context of cardiac failure or cardiogenic shock, it is termed 'secondary'. Successful defibrillation is less likely in secondary ventricular fibrillation.

Ventricular fibrillation can occur without myocardial infarction in patients with severe coronary artery disease and may be the first clinical

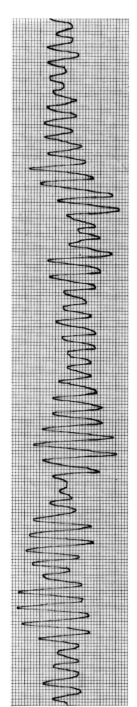

*Fig.* 11.1. Ventricular fibrillation.

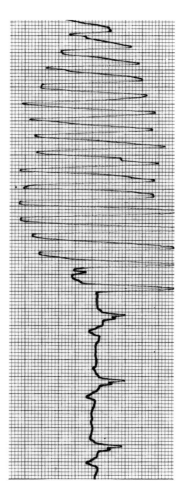

*Fig.* 11.2 Ventricular ectopic beat initiating ventricular fibrillation.

manifestation of the disease. Ventricular fibrillation can occur in other cardiac disorders but is discussed in this chapter because primary ventricular fibrillation due to myocardial infarction is a major cause of death in the Western world.

Rarely ventricular fibrillation is a brief event, spontaneously reverting to normal rhythm. Otherwise, without prompt treatment, irreversible cerebral and myocardial damage will quickly develop.

### Treatment

Occasionally a praecordial blow is effective. Usually defibrillation is necessary (*see* Chapter 14). On a coronary care unit a defibrillator should be immediately available so that little or no time need be spent on cardio-pulmonary resuscitation. Though cardiac massage has been shown to sustain an adequate cerebral circulation for periods of 20 min and more, the low arterial pressure during massage will lead to poor myocardial perfusion and consequent extension of the size of myocardial infarction unless normal rhythm can be restored very quickly.

Successful defibrillation can be achieved with a 200 Ws (Joules) DC shock in 90 per cent of cases. If unsuccessful, a second shock at the same energy level is sometimes effective, although it is probably best to increase the energy of a further shock to 300 or 400 Ws. The treatment of resistant ventricular fibrillation is discussed in Chapter 14.

Once normal rhythm is restored, lignocaine (or second-line drug if lignocaine has been found to be ineffective) should be given quickly to prevent further ventricular fibrillation though it has to be said there is little evidence to show that lignocaine or other anti-arrhythmic drugs are effective in this situation.

### VENTRICULAR FLUTTER

Ventricular flutter is a very fast ventricular rhythm in which there are rapid, continuous changes in waveform, distinction between QRS complexes and T waves being impossible (*Fig.* 11.3). For practical purposes, it is the same as ventricular fibrillation.

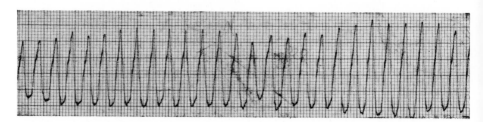

*Fig.* 11.3. Ventricular flutter.

## PREVENTION OF VENTRICULAR FIBRILLATION

Conventional teaching is that ventricular fibrillation and tachycardia are heralded by ventricular ectopic beats which are frequent, multifocal, 'R on T', or are repetitive – the 'warning arrhythmias' (*Figs.* 11.4–11.7). It is common practice to suppress these ectopic beats with anti-arrhythmic agents, usually lignocaine, in the hope that ventricular fibrillation will be prevented.

However, the significance of warning arrhythmias and the value of their suppression has been questioned. Analysis of continuous ECG recordings has demonstrated that ventricular ectopic beats occur in virtually all cases of acute infarction and that warning arrhythmias are as common in patients who do not develop ventricular fibrillation as in those who do. Furthermore, there is evidence to show that ventricular fibrillation may not be preceded by warning arrhythmias and that when these do occur, staff in even the best coronary care units often fail to detect them.

It is disappointing that, in spite of 20 years of development in coronary care, there is no clear approach to the prevention of ventricular fibrillation. Until the situation is clarified by further studies, one of two policies can be adopted:

1. *Prophylaxis for all patients with acute infarction.* This approach has been quite widely advocated on the grounds that since 'warning arrhythmias' do not in fact warn, lignocaine should be given to all patients with definite or suspected acute infarction. However, a consistently

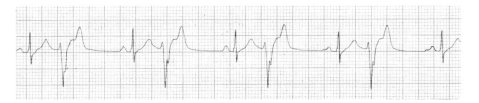

*Fig.* 11.4. Frequent unifocal ventricular ectopic beats.

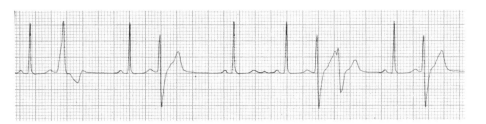

*Fig.* 11.5. Frequent multifocal ventricular ectopic beats. The first ectopic beat arises from a different focus from that of subsequent ectopic beats. There is a couplet of ectopic beats after the fourth sinus beat.

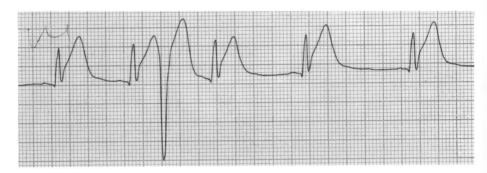

*Fig.* 11.6. Interpolated 'R on T' ventricular ectopic beat.

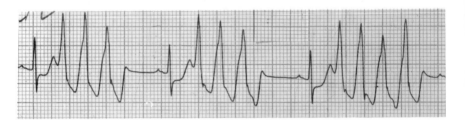

*Fig.* 11.7. Salvoes of ventricular ectopic beats, initiated by 'R on T' ectopics.

therapeutic plasma level of the drug is required. In order to achieve this, quite complex regimens of administration are necessary which may be impracticable for many busy coronary care units. Furthermore, with the high dosages of lignocaine that are required, side effects due to lignocaine toxicity are frequent. Recently, it has been suggested that high doses of lignocaine may reduce the incidence of ventricular fibrillation only at the expense of a higher incidence of asystole. Reports vary as to whether lignocaine does actually reduce the incidence of ventricular fibrillation. With the possible exception of intravenous beta-blocking drugs, there are no reports of other drugs being of prophylactic value.

2. *No prophylaxis.* Since only a minority of patients develops ventricular fibrillation, some (including the author) advocate no prophylaxis provided trained staff are immediately available to defibrillate if ventricular fibrillation does occur. However, there are two reservations about this approach. First, occasionally it is not possible to resuscitate a patient with primary ventricular fibrillation. Secondly, though it is widely believed that the prognosis following correction of primary ventricular fibrillation is normal, there are a few reports suggesting that it may in fact be impaired.

*Long-term Therapy after Ventricular Fibrillation or Tachycardia?*

If the above arrhythmias occur within the first 24 hours of acute infarction, they are unlikely to recur after discharge from the coronary care unit and there is no need to prescribe oral anti-arrhythmic therapy. On the other hand, when these arrhythmias occur after the first 24 hours, there is usually extensive myocardial damage and recurrence is likely. In this situation oral therapy should be given for several months and in-hospital and ambulatory ECG monitoring should be carried out to ensure that whatever has been prescribed is effective.

## VENTRICULAR TACHYCARDIA

Ventricular tachycardia may be self-terminating (*Fig.* 11.7) or sustained (*Fig.* 11.8). Ventricular tachycardia may be initiated by either 'R on T' or late ventricular ectopic beats (*Fig.* 11.9).

Sometimes ventricular tachycardia will severely impair cardiac function and result in shock or circulatory arrest. On the other hand, ventricular tachycardia may cause few or no symptoms. It must be emphasized that in myocardial infarction a regular tachycardia with broad ventricular complexes is usually ventricular in origin, even in the absence of haemo-dynamic deterioration (*see* Chapter 8).

### Treatment

If cardiac arrest or shock occurs, immediate synchronized DC countershock is indicated. Otherwise intravenous lignocaine should be given. If lignocaine fails, second-line drugs include mexiletine, disopyramide, flecainide and amiodarone (*see* Chapter 12). Overdrive ventricular pacing should be considered in recurrent ventricular tachycardia or when a pacing wire is already in place for the treatment of a conduction disorder.

## IDIOVENTRICULAR TACHYCARDIA

Idioventricular tachycardia, also referred to as accelerated ventricular rhythm or 'slow' ventricular tachycardia, is usually benign and treatment is not indicated (*Fig.* 11.10). Rarely, acceleration of the rate can occur, necessitating treatment.

## ATRIAL ECTOPIC BEATS

Occasional atrial ectopic beats can be ignored: however, frequent atrial ectopic beats often herald atrial fibrillation. It is best to digitalize the patient so that, should atrial fibrillation occur, the ventricular rate will be controlled.

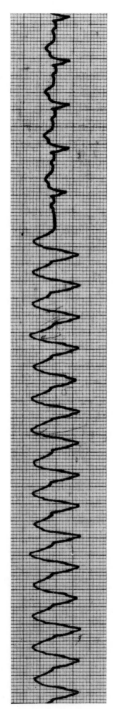

*Fig.* 11.8. Ventricular tachycardia, terminated by mexiletine.

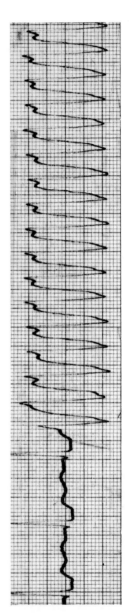

*Fig.* 11.9. Ventricular tachycardia initiated by 'R on T' ectopic beat.

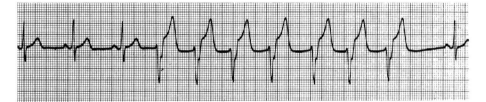

*Fig*. 11.10. Idioventricular tachycardia.

## ATRIAL FIBRILLATION

In atrial fibrillation, the resultant rapid ventricular rate and loss of atrial contribution to ventricular filling can sometimes cause severe hypotension or heart failure (*Fig*. 11.11). In either situation, cardioversion is necessary; otherwise, the ventricular rate should be slowed by verapamil or digoxin. Spontaneous reversion to sinus rhythm is quite common.

Sustained atrial fibrillation usually indicates extensive myocardial damage and hence a poor long-term prognosis. Often left ventricular failure will be present and necessitate diuretic therapy.

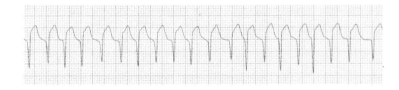

*Fig*. 11.11. Atrial fibrillation with rapid ventricular rate in anterior infarction (lead V3).

## PAROXYSMAL SUPRAVENTRICULAR TACHYCARDIA

Paroxysmal (i.e. AV re-entrant) supraventricular tachycardia can only occur if there is an additional AV connection, either bypassing or within the AV node (*see* Chapter 6). Thus, paroxysmal supraventricular tachycardia is unlikely to occur for the first time during acute myocardial infarction. When supraventricular tachycardia is diagnosed in a patient with acute infarction the correct diagnosis is usually atrial flutter, atrial fibrillation or even ventricular tachycardia.

## ATRIAL FLUTTER

The diagnostic features are discussed in Chapter 6. Usually 2 : 1 AV block occurs. Intravenous verapamil is useful, in that it will slow the ventricular rate and may occasionally effect a return to sinus rhythm. Low energy DC countershock or rapid atrial pacing are often necessary for a prompt return to normal rhythm. Digoxin is best avoided because even large doses may not control the ventricular rate and will be a contra-indication to cardioversion.

## SINUS AND JUNCTIONAL BRADYCARDIAS

Sinus and junctional bradycardias are common, particularly in inferior infarction (*Figs.* 11.12, 11.13). If uncomplicated, no treatment is required. Bradycardia may be beneficial in acute infarction, in that myocardial oxygen consumption is related to heart rate and a low oxygen consumption might limit infarct size.

However, if bradycardia is associated with signs of a low cardiac output such as hypotension (systolic blood pressure less than 90 mmHg), mental confusion, oliguria, cold peripheries or ventricular arrhythmias, intravenous atropine (initially 0·3 to 0·6 mg) should be given. Temporary cardiac pacing is occasionally necessary and is preferable to frequent doses of atropine.

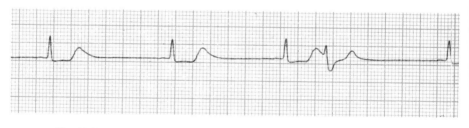

*Fig.* 11.12. Sinus bradycardia. The fourth beat is an 'R on T' ventricular ectopic.

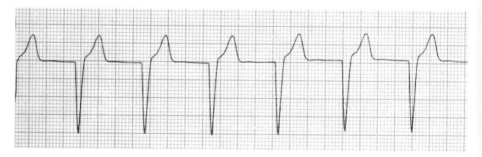

*Fig.* 11.13. Junctional escape rhythm as a result of sinus bradycardia in anterior infarction (lead V4).

## AV BLOCK

The management and prognosis of AV block in inferior and anterior infarction differ markedly.

### Inferior Infarction

In inferior infarction AV block is common and is due to ischaemia of the AV node. Recovery of AV node function usually occurs within a few days although sometimes it takes up to 3 weeks. Permanent AV node damage is very rare. The prognosis for inferior infarction complicated by AV block is good.

First degree and Mobitz type I second degree (Wenkebach) AV block (*Figs.* 11.14, 11.15) require no treatment, although drugs that may worsen AV node function, e.g. digoxin and verapamil should be avoided.

If complete block develops (*Fig.* 11.16), subsidiary pacemakers in the bundle of His control the ventricular rate. These pacemakers usually

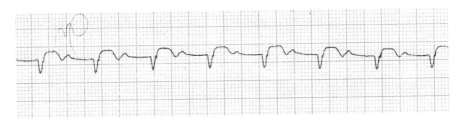

*Fig.* 11.14. First degree AV block (lead AVF).

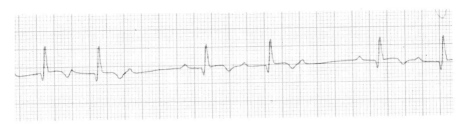

*Fig.* 11.15. Wenkebach AV block in inferior infarction (lead AVF).

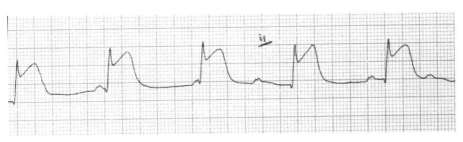

*Fig.* 11.16. Inferior infarction complicated by complete AV block (lead II).

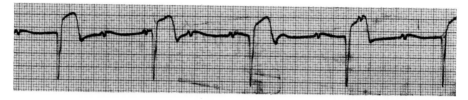

*Fig.* 11.17. Complete heart block with ventricular rate of 38/min.

discharge at a fairly high rate and are reliable. Thus, asystole and symptoms resulting from a low ventricular rate are unusual.

Only rarely does the ventricular rate fall very low (less than 40/min), when Stokes—Adams attacks are likely to occur or complications from a low ventricular rate such as heart failure, hypotension, mental confusion, oliguria and ventricular arrhythmias may result (*Fig.* 11.17). In these cicumstances temporary cardiac pacing is necessary. There is no place for steroids or catecholamines in an attempt to improve AV node function, although in the first couple of hours after infarction, atropine may be effective.

### Anterior Infarction

In anterior infarction it is the bundle branches rather than the AV node which are usually the site of ischaemic damage. AV block is more serious than in inferior infarction for two reasons. First, the subsidiary pacemakers which arise below the level of the block in the distal specialized conducting system tend to be much slower and less reliable. Thus, circulatory disturbances due to a low ventricular rate are common and ventricular standstill frequently occurs. Secondly, an extensive area of infarction is required to affect both bundle branches. Prognosis after myocardial infarction is related to the extent of infarction and is thus poor in patients with anterior infarction complicated by AV block.

Evidence of bilateral bundle branch damage (alternating right and left

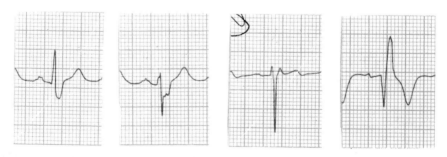

*Fig.* 11.18. Left anterior fascicular and right bundle branch block in anterior infarction (leads I, II, III and V1).

bundle branch block, or right bundle branch block with left anterior or posterior hemiblock) usually precedes the onset of second degree (Mobitz type II) or complete AV block (*Figs.* 11.18–11.21). The chance of bilateral bundle branch damage progressing to second degree or complete heart block is approximately 30 per cent. The first manifestation of these higher degrees of block may be ventricular standstill (*Fig.* 11.22). For this

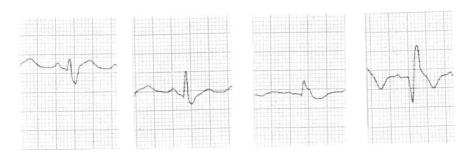

*Fig.* 11.19. Left posterior fascicular and right bundle branch block in anterior infarction (leads I, II, III and V1).

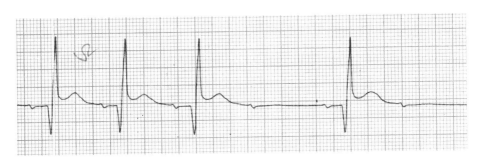

*Fig.* 11.20. Intermittent Mobitz type II AV block in a patient with bifascicular block due to anterior infarction (lead V2).

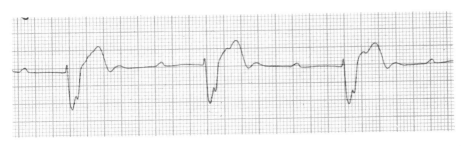

*Fig.* 11.21. Complete AV block in a patient with anterior myocardial infarction. Because the atrial rate is twice the ventricular rate, at first glance in this short rhythm strip it appears that there is 2 : 1 AV block. However, measurement of the PR intervals indicates that they are not constant.

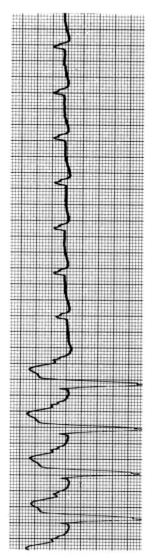

*Fig.* 11.22. Sudden development of complete AV block in a patient with bifascicular block due to anterior infarction. Following four ventricular beats, there is asystole — only atrial activity is seen.

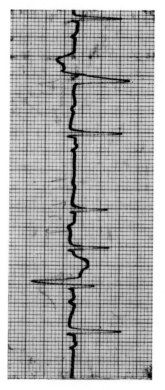

*Fig.* 11.23. Modified V1 lead using three chest electrodes. Atrial ectopic beats conducted with right bundle branch block, normal intraventricular conduction and left bundle branch block can be seen.

reason a temporary transvenous pacemaker should be inserted when there is evidence of bilateral bundle branch damage even though the patient is in sinus rhythm.

Second and third degree AV block in anterior infarction are unlikely to be uncomplicated and are therefore always an indication for temporary cardiac pacing. Sinus rhythm normally returns within a few days but evidence of bundle branch damage usually persists. Complete AV block can recur in the weeks or months after acute infarction and is one of the causes of sudden death in this group of patients. There is, however, no conclusive evidence to show that implantation of a permanent pacemaker will improve the prognosis. This is because many of these patients will have extensive infarction with consequent risk of death due to ventricular fibrillation or heart failure. There are, however, some patients where clinical evidence, such as a relatively low rise in cardiac enzymes and absence of cardiac failure, suggests that the infarct may not be large. In these patients, particularly the younger ones, implantation of a permanent pacemaker should be considered.

## AV DISSOCIATION

In contrast to complete AV block, in AV dissociation the atrial rate is lower than the ventricular rate and no treatment is necessary.

## ELECTRODE PLACEMENT FOR MONITORING

Detection of atrial activity during an arrhythmia is often the key to the diagnosis. Chest electrodes for monitoring the ECG should be so placed that atrial activity can be clearly seen.

Lead V1 often shows atrial activity most clearly but is impracticable for continuous monitoring. A modifed V1 lead can be achieved with three chest electrodes by placing the positive electrode over the fourth inter-space at the right sternal edge, the negative electrode beneath the outer quarter of the left clavicle and the earth electrode beneath the outer quarter of the right clavicle. Not only will this lead system clearly show atrial activity, but it will allow distinction between beats having right and left bundle branch block appearance (*Fig.* 11.23). In some patients, however, the lead system is not suitable because the ventricular complexes in lead V1 are of too small an amplitude.

## Main Points

1. Ventricular fibrillation occurs during the first hour of acute myo-cardial infarction in more than 30 per cent of patients: the incidence falls progressively thereafter.

2. Frequent, 'R on T' and other 'warning arrhythmias' are very common in acute infarction and are not predictive of ventricular

fibrillation. Suppression by anti-arrhythmic drugs is not indicated.

**3.** Immediate defibrillation should be carried out if ventricular fibrillation occurs.

**4.** Ventricular fibrillation or other major ventricular arrhythmia during the first 24 hours of infarction is not an indication for long-term anti-arrhythmic therapy whereas therapy should be given if these arrhythmias occur after 24 hours.

**5.** Atrial fibrillation and ventricular arrhythmias arising 24 hours or more after acute infarction are usually associated with extensive myocardial damage and hence an impaired prognosis.

**6.** Sinus and junctional bradycardia and complete AV block due to inferior infarction do not require treatment unless there are symptoms, marked hypotension, other signs of shock or ventricular arrhythmias.

**7.** AV block due to acute inferior infarction may persist for up to three weeks and is very rarely an indication for permanent pacemaker implantation.

**8.** In acute anterior infarction, a temporary pacemaker should always be inserted if there is second or third degree AV block or evidence of bilateral bundle branch damage. These conduction disturbances in the setting of anterior infarction imply extensive myocardial damage.

# Chapter 12

# Anti-arrhythmic Drugs

Drugs are the mainstay of treatment for arrhythmias but their limitations should be appreciated. First, anti-arrhythmic drugs are of limited efficacy: in other words a drug prescribed in the correct dose for an appropriate indication will not infrequently fail to work. Secondly, unwanted effects often occur. The most common are symptoms from the gastrointestinal and central nervous systems, hypotension, heart failure and impairment of the specialized cardiac conducting tissues. Occasionally, drugs may be 'pro-arrhythmic' in that they may cause or worsen arrhythmias. Thirdly, with many drugs it can be difficult to maintain therapeutic drug levels. Fourthly, though some insight into the mode of action of these drugs has been gained, selection for an individual patient of a drug that is both effective and well tolerated is often a process of trial and error.

It should be remembered that drugs are only one form of treatment and that in some situations other approaches such as vagal stimulation, cardioversion, artificial pacing or surgery may be more appropriate. A number of factors may influence the choice of treatment: the type of arrhythmia, the urgency of the situation, the need for short or long-term therapy, and the presence of impaired myocardial performance, sinus node dysfunction or abnormal AV conduction.

It is important to bear in mind the purpose for which an anti-arrhythmic drug is being given. In some situations, a drug is given to terminate an arrhythmia while in others the purpose is prevention of recurrence of an arrhythmia. Though it would seem reasonable to assume that the oral preparation of a drug that has terminated an arrhythmia when given intravenously would be successful in preventing its recurrence, this is often not the case in practice. Generally, drugs are better at terminating arrhythmias than at preventing recurrence. Sometimes, the aim of anti-arrhythmic therapy is to slow the heart rate during an arrhythmia rather than to restore sinus rhythm.

## MODES OF ACTION

The modes of action of anti-arrhythmic drugs can be classified in two ways: according to their effects in the intact heart and according to their effects at cellular level as established by *in vitro* studies. The latter classification is of very limited clinical value. Even though this book is concerned with the practical aspects of arrhythmia treatment, this classification is described because it is referred to widely.

## Clinical Classification

Drugs are divided into three groups according to their main site or sites of action in the intact heart (Table 12.1). The first group consists of drugs whose chief action is to slow conduction in the AV node. These drugs are therefore useful in the treatment of arrhythmias of supraventricular origin but are of little or no use in the treatment of ventricular arrhythmias.

*Table* 12.1.  Classification of anti-arrhythmic actions according to their principal site(s) of action in the intact heart

---

*AV node*
  Verapamil, Diltiazem, Digoxin, Beta-Blockers

*Ventricles*
  Lignocaine, mexiletine, tocainide, phenytoin

*Atria, ventricles and bundle of Kent*
  Quinidine, disopyramide, amiodarone, flecainide, procainamide

---

In the second group, there are drugs that work mainly in ventricular arrhythmias. The third group comprises drugs that act on the atria, ventricles and, in cases of Wolff–Parkinson–White syndrome, the bundle of Kent. Thus, they may be useful in both supraventricular and ventricular arrhythmias.

## Action Potential Classification

In this classification, drugs are divided into four main classes depending upon their electrophysiological effects at cellular level (Table 12.2).

Class I drugs impede the transport of sodium across the cell membrane during the initiation of cellular activation and thereby reduce the rate of rise of the action potential (phase 0). Many drugs fall into this group. They have been subdivided into classes A, B and C according to their effect on the duration of the action potential (which is reflected in the surface electrocardiogram by the QT interval).

1A drugs increase the duration, 1B drugs shorten it and 1C drugs have little effect. The anti-arrhythmic action of 1B drugs is confined to the ventricles whereas 1A and 1C drugs affect both atria and ventricles. 1A and particularly 1C drugs slow intraventricular conduction.

*Table* 12.2. Examples of action potential classification

|   | [I] | [II] | [III] | [IV] |
|---|-----|------|-------|------|
| A | Quinidine<br>Procainamide<br>Disopyramide | Beta blockers<br>Bretylium | Amiodarone<br>Sotalol<br>Bretylium | Verapamil<br>Diltiazem |
| B | Lignocaine<br>Mexiletine<br>Tocainide<br>Phenytoin<br>Aprindine<br>Ethmozine<br>Propafenone | | | |
| C | Flecainide<br>Encainide<br>Lorcainide | | | |

Class II drugs interfere with the effects of the sympathetic nervous system on the heart. They do not affect the action potential of most myocardial cells but do reduce the slope of spontaneous depolarization (phase 4) of cells with pacemaker activity and thus the rate of pacemaker discharge.

Class III drugs prolong the duration of the action potential and hence the length of the refractory period, but do not slow phase 0.

Class IV drugs antagonise the transport of calcium across the cell membrane which follows the inward flux of sodium during cellular activation. Cells in the AV and sinus nodes are particularly susceptible. It should be noted that some calcium antagonists, e.g. nifedipine, do not have an anti-arrhythmic action.

It can be seen from Table 12.2 that the majority of drugs are in class I, several drugs have more than one class of action, and drugs within class I differ significantly in their clinical effects.

## NOTES ON INDIVIDUAL DRUGS

### Lignocaine

Lignocaine is the first-line drug for ventricular arrhythmias but is ineffective in arrhythmias of supraventricular origin. The drug is a vasoconstrictor and, unlike many drugs, rarely causes hypotension or heart failure.

A 100 mg bolus given intravenously over 2 min will usually be effective. If unsuccessful, a further bolus (50–75 mg) should be given after 5 min. It should be noted that there are several concentrations of lignocaine available and occasional disasters have occurred because the wrong concentration has been used. For example, with 1 per cent lignocaine, 10 ml contains 100 mg.

Lignocaine is often used for short-term prophylaxis of ventricular arrhythmias. The therapeutic effect of lignocaine is closely related to plasma levels, which fall rapidly after a bolus injection. Thus it is necessary to give a continuous infusion immediately after the bolus. There is, however, no point in giving a continuous infusion if the bolus has failed to work or, since lignocaine cannot be administered orally, if long-term prophylaxis is required.

It can be difficult to maintain therapeutic levels of lignocaine. With sub-therapeutic levels, the patient is at risk from arrhythmias while toxic levels may cause symptoms related to the central nervous system, including light-headedness, confusion, twitching, paraesthesiae and epileptic fits. With conventional infusion rates (1–4 mg/min) sub-therapeutic levels commonly occur in the first hour or two after the infusion is commenced. A number of fairly complex regimens have been developed to avoid this problem, though they may be too complex for routine use and do increase the risk of toxicity:

75 mg i.v. bolus plus infusion at 10 mg/min for 20 min, reducing to 1·5 mg/min.
25 mg/min up to total dose of 200–300 mg depending on body weight, followed by 2–3 mg/min.
Two 100 mg boluses separated by 10 min followed by infusion at 2–4 mg/min.

Lignocaine is metabolized by the liver, and where there is liver disease or where hepatic blood flow is reduced by heart failure or by shock, dosages should be halved to avoid toxicity. Hypokalaemia may impair lignocaine's efficacy.

## Mexiletine

Mexiletine is very similar to lignocaine in its therapeutic and haemo-dynamic actions but it can be given orally as well as parenterally. There is a narrow margin between therapeutic and toxic effects and symptoms due to toxicity, such as nausea, vomiting, confusion, tremor, ataxia, as well as bradycardia and hypotension, are not uncommon.

Intravenously, the drug is given in a dose of 100–250 mg over 5–10 min, followed by 250 mg over 1 h and a further 250 mg over 2 h. The infusion can then be continued at 0·5–1·0 mg/min or oral therapy started.

The oral dose is 200–300 mg 8-hourly. If the patient has not received a prior infusion, a loading dose of 400 mg can be given. Up to one-third of patients experience unwanted effects with long-term administration.

The drug is mainly metabolized by the liver and doses should be reduced if there is hepatic disease or heart failure. Approximately 10 per cent is excreted unchanged in the urine. Renal excretion is inhibited by alkaline urine but this is not a problem in practice.

## Tocainide

Tocainide is also similar to lignocaine. Like mexiletine it is effective both intravenously and orally. Its duration of action is somewhat longer than mexiletine, making twice daily oral administration possible. Forty per cent of the drug is excreted by the kidneys and dosage should be reduced if there is renal impairment.

The intravenous dosage is 750 mg over 15 min. The daily oral dosage is 1200 mg. Side effects include tremor, light-headedness, confusion and convulsions.

## Quinidine

Quinidine can be effective in both supraventricular and ventricular arrhythmias. The drug is rarely used parenterally because severe hypotension may result. Orally, its use has been limited because of its reputation for causing dangerous rhythm disturbances, especially torsade de pointes tachycardia. However, slow-release preparations (e.g. Kinidin Durules) enable therapeutic levels to be maintained with much less risk of toxicity and have the advantage that twice-daily administration (0·5–0·75 g twice-daily) is sufficient.

Impaired sinus node and myocardial function are less likely to be worsened by quinidine than by disopyramide or beta-blockers. Because it has a mild anticholinergic action, AV node conduction may be enhanced with a resultant increase in ventricular rate during atrial flutter and fibrillation.

QT interval prolongation occurs with therapeutic doses, but lengthening of the QRS complex by more than 25 per cent indicates toxicity. The drug should not be given to patients whose QT interval is already prolonged. Gastrointestinal symptoms are not infrequent. Tinnitus, deafness, thrombocytopenia and hypotension occasionally occur. Quinidine therapy can elevate digoxin levels and precipitate toxicity. The drug is metabolized by the liver and doses should be reduced if there is hepatic disease.

## Procainamide

Procainamide has similar anti-arrhythmic properties to quinidine. It is not widely used nowadays. It has a short half-life necessitating very frequent dosage when given orally. Even with a slow release preparation, 8-hourly administration is necessary. Furthermore, unwanted effects such as systemic lupus syndrome, gastrointestinal symptoms, hypotension and agranulocytosis make it unsuitable for long-term use. Impaired renal function and a slow acetylator status both reduce procainamide requirements.

N-acetyl-procainamide, a metabolite of procainamide, has been shown to have a longer duration of action and not to cause systemic lupus.

## Disopyramide

Disopyramide is widely used for both supraventricular and ventricular arrhythmias. However, it is only moderately effective and does have significant unwanted effects.

The intravenous dose is 1·5–2·0 mg/kg up to a maximum of 150 mg, given over no less than 5 min. The injection should be stopped if the arrhythmia is terminated. Therapy can be continued by intravenous infusion at 20–30 mg/h up to a maximum of 800 mg daily or the patient can be transferred to oral therapy. The oral dose is 300–800 mg daily in three or four divided doses. If necessary a loading dose of 300 mg can be given.

Given intravenously, the drug is more likely to cause hypotension and heart failure than lignocaine and related drugs and its use can be disastrous if the recommended minimum period of administration is ignored.

Orally, the drug's side effects are mainly related to its anticholinergic (atropine-like) action which often causes a dry mouth, blurred vision, urinary hesitancy or retention and, by enhancing AV nodal conduction, an increase in the ventricular response to atrial flutter and fibrillation. The drug may precipitate heart failure in patients with impaired myocardial function. It may occasionally induce torsade de pointes tachycardia and should not be given to patients with QT interval prolongation. Disopyramide may worsen impaired sinus node function and is contraindicated in the sick sinus syndrome. The drug is partially excreted by the kidneys and dosage should be reduced in renal disease.

## Flecainide

Flecainide is a potent drug which can be given both orally and parenterally. Its indications include ventricular arrhythmias and pre-excitation syndromes.

It has a long half-life of approximately 16 hours. The intravenous dose is 2 mg/kg body weight over not less than 10 min and, because the drug has a significant negative inotropic effect, it should be given more slowly in patients with poor ventricular function. Orally, the dosage is 100–200 mg b.d. After 3–5 days it may be possible to reduce the dose.

The drug has a narrow therapeutic range and it may be difficult to achieve therapeutic action without unwanted effects. The most common side effect is visual disturbance, particularly on rotating the head. Light-headedness and nausea can also occur. The drug can increase the endocardial pacing threshold.

Flecainide causes slight prolongation of the QRS complex and hence the QT interval: it does not prolong the JT component of the QT interval as does quinidine and disopyramide. There are a number of reports of the drug causing serious ventricular arrhythmias.

## Amiodarone

This drug has several advantages over other drugs. It is highly effective in both supraventricular and ventricular rhythm disorders: even in arrhythmias refractory to other drugs there is a 70 per cent success rate. It has a remarkably long half-life (20–100 days), so that the drug need only be given once daily or even less frequently. It does not significantly impair ventricular performance and can be given to patients in heart failure.

However, it has important unwanted effects which point to the long-term use of amiodarone being confined to patients with arrhythmias that are dangerous or resistant to other drugs, or where the risk of side effects is not a major consideration because the patient's prognosis is poor, e.g. the elderly and those with severe myocardial damage.

Orally, the drug has a delayed onset of action. It usually takes 3–7 days before it takes effect and it may take 50 days to reach its maximal action. When necessary, delay can be minimized by giving large doses, e.g. 1200 mg for 1 or 2 weeks. The dose can then be reduced to 400–600 mg daily. Once it is established that the drug is effective, it is recommended that the dose be progressively reduced until the lowest effective dose is found. Some patients need as little as 200 mg on alternate days. However, in the case of dangerous arrhythmias, it is best not to reduce the dose beneath 400 mg daily.

Intravenous administration will lead to an earlier effect but, unlike most drugs, an immediate anti-arrhythmic action rarely occurs: an effect is usually seen within 1–24 hours. In patients with arrhythmias which have been difficult to control, it is often worth resorting to intravenous amiodarone in spite of the delay in action rather than try other less effective drugs which are usually associated with a higher risk of acute side effects.

The recommended intravenous dosage is 5 mg/kg body weight over 30 min to 1 h followed by 15 mg/kg over 24 h. In an emergency the initial infusion can be given more rapidly – at the risk of marked hypotension. The drug should be given via a central venous line to avoid phlebitis. If this is not possible, frequent change of site of peripheral infusion will usually be sufficient.

The most common long term unwanted effects are corneal micro-deposits and skin photosensitivity. Corneal microdeposits develop in virtually all patients but ocular damage does not occur. These micro-deposits disappear if the drug is stopped and are a useful sign of compliance. Skin photosensitivity to UV–A radiation affects over 30 per cent of patients and is the commonest reason for stopping the drug: it may persist for over a year afterwards. Though only a minority experience severe photosensitivity, all patients should be warned about the possibility.

The drug potentiates both digoxin and oral anticoagulants. Amiodarone contains iodine and causes elevation of both serum thyroxine and reversed tri-iodothyronine, and depression of serum tri-iodothyronine, the patient remaining euthyroid. However, hypothyroidism and hyperthyroidism do occasionally occur. If the latter develops, serum thyroxine will be low and TSH will be elevated. The biochemical diagnosis of hyperthyroidism is not so easy and more reliance must be placed on clinical signs.

Nausea, alopecia, rash, blue–grey skin pigmentation, tremor and nightmares can occur. More serious, but fairly rare side effects, include pulmonary fibrosis, neuropathy, myopathy and hepatitis. The drug's class III action results in QT prolongation, often with prominent U waves. There are a few reports of the drug causing torsade de pointes tachycardia.

## Verapamil

Intravenous verapamil (5–10 mg over 30–60 s) quickly and effectively slows AV nodal conduction. It is the drug of choice for the termination of paroxysmal (AV re-entrant) supraventricular tachycardia. It will promptly slow the ventricular response to atrial fibrillation and flutter and in a minority of cases, in addition to its action on the AV node, may actually restore sinus rhythm.

Orally, verapamil is less effective and because much of each dose is metabolized by the liver, large doses (40–120 mg t.d.s.) are required. Oral verapamil is rarely useful alone but is very useful in combination with digoxin in controlling the ventricular response to atrial fibrillation. If this cannot be achieved by apparently adequate doses of digoxin alone. Serum digoxin levels are in fact elevated by moderately large doses of verapamil.

Intravenous verapamil is contraindicated if the patient has received an intravenous or oral beta-blocker. Profound bradycardia or hypotension can result and may be fatal. Sometimes, the combination of oral verapamil and a beta-blocker will cause profound sinus or junctional bradycardia. Verapamil is contraindicated in patients with impaired sinus or atrioventricular node function or digoxin toxicity unless a ventricular pacing wire is in situ because of its depressant effects on the sinus and AV nodes.

## Beta-adrenoceptor Antagonists

These drugs have anti-arrhythmic properties by virtue of their principal action – antagonizing the effects of catecholamines on the heart. They are most effective in arrhythmias caused by increased sympathetic nervous system activity, e.g. those caused by exertion, emotion, thyrotoxicosis, acute myocardial infarction and the hereditary QT prolongation syndromes.

Beta-blocking drugs slow AV nodal conduction and thus, like verapamil, are useful in arrhythmias of supraventricular origin. However, they are less often successful than verapamil, and, since the latter drug cannot be safely administered once beta-blockers have been given, verapamil is the treatment of choice. Unwanted bradycardia caused by beta-blockade can usually quickly be reversed by atropine.

Sotalol, in addition to its beta-blocking property, prolongs the duration of the action potential and hence QT interval: it has a significant class III, or amiodarone-like action. Unlike other beta-blockers, sotalol has a marked effect upon the recovery periods of atrial and ventricular myocardium and accessory AV pathways. Sotalol is more effective than other beta-blockers for prevention of supraventricular arrhythmias and may possibly be of value for ventricular arrhythmias. There are a few reports of high doses of the drug—usually in association with other drugs or hypokalaemia—of causing torsade de pointes tachycardia. The oral dosage is 160–320 mg daily.

## Digoxin

The main use of digoxin is an AV nodal blocking drug in the control of the ventricular rate during atrial fibrillation. The usual dose is 0.25–0.375 mg daily. A number of factors, e.g. hypokalaemia, renal impairment, dehydration (often caused by diuretics) and therapy with quinidine, verapamil or amiodarone, predispose to digoxin toxicity and are an indication for dosage reduction. Digoxin toxicity is discussed in Chapter 17.

## Therapeutic Range of Plasma Levels

The therapeutic plasma levels of the commonly used anti-arrhythmic drugs are given in Table 12.3. However, it should be appreciated that

*Table* 12.3. Therapeutic range of plasma levels for some anti-arrhythmic drugs

| | | |
|---|---|---|
| Lignocaine | 1.4–6.0 | µg/ml |
| Mexiletine | 0.5–2.0 | µg/ml |
| Tocainide | 6.0–12.0 | µg/ml |
| Quinidine | 2.3–5.0 | µg/ml |
| Procainamide | 4.0–10.0 | µg/ml |
| Disopyramide | 2.0–6.0 | µg/ml |
| Flecainide | 200–1000 | ng/ml |
| Verapamil | 100–200 | µg/ml |

measurement of plasma levels is of limited use and is not often necessary in routine treatment.

If there is good objective evidence of a therapeutic effect with a conventional dosage regimen and there are no unwanted effects, measurement of a drug's plasma level is of little importance. However, knowledge of a drug's level can be helpful with some clinical problems, e.g. when there is doubt as to whether a patient is taking his therapy.

# Main Points

1. Anti-arrhythmic drugs are of limited efficacy and often cause unwanted effects.

2. Choice of anti-arrhythmic therapy should be tailored to the individual patient and depends on the arrhythmia, the degree of associated circulatory disturbance, the presence of impaired myocardial, sinus node or AV node function, need for short or long-term treatment and concurrent administration of other drugs.

3. Drugs are usually better at terminating arrhythmias than at preventing their recurrence.

4. Intravenous verapamil should not be given to a patient who has received a beta-blocker.

5. Disopyramide, flecainide and beta-blockers have a marked negative inotropic action and may precipitate heart failure in patients with extensive myocardial damage.

6. Intravenous verapamil is the drug of choice for the acute control of arrhythmias of supraventricular origin.

7. Lignocaine is the first-line drug for termination of ventricular tachycardia.

8. Amiodarone is the most effective anti-arrhythmic agent currently available but its long term use should be confined to the treatment of patients with arrhythmias that are dangerous or are refractory to other forms of treatment, or who have a poor prognosis.

# Chapter 13

# Cardioversion

Cardioversion is the use of an electric shock of high energy and brief duration to terminate a tachyarrhythmia. The shock, which is usually delivered by two electrodes placed on the chest wall, depolarizes the myocardium thus interrupting the tachycardia and allowing the sinus node to resume control of the heart rhythm.

## PROCEDURE

Facilities for monitoring the ECG and for cardiopulmonary resuscitation must be available. The rhythm should be checked immediately prior to cardioversion to ensure that spontaneous reversion has not occurred.

### Anaesthesia

Cardioversion is painful, causing involuntary contraction of the chest wall and upper limb girdle muscles. A conscious patient should be given a short-acting anaesthetic, e.g. methohexitone or at least an amnesic agent, e.g. intravenous diazepam (5–20 mg). The patient should fast for 6 h before elective cardioversion, though this will not be possible in an emergency.

### Delivery of Shock

The shock is delivered by means of two electrode paddles placed on the chest wall, positioned so that the heart lies between them. Usually one electrode is placed over the cardiac apex and the other to the right of the upper sternum. Alternatively, if a flat paddle is available this can be placed beneath the patient's back, behind the heart, and the second paddle positioned anteriorly over the praecordium.

To achieve good electrical contact and to avoid burning the skin, electrode jelly must be generously applied to the areas beneath the paddles. However, it is essential to avoid spreading jelly between the two paddles. Recently, pads impregnated with electrode gel have been introduced, with the advantage that they avoid the spreading of jelly over unwanted areas, including the operator!

The defibrillator is charged to the desired energy level (*see below*), which takes a few seconds. The charge is usually released by pressing the button(s) on the defibrillator paddle(s). Application of the paddles with firm pressure reduces the electrical resistance of the thorax. Just before discharge it is essential to ensure that no one is in contact with the patient or the patient's bed.

If cardioversion is unsuccessful, depending on the circumstances, further shocks with higher energy levels may be tried. The heart rhythm should usually be monitored for some hours after cardioversion.

### Synchronization

Ventricular fibrillation may be induced if a shock coincides with the ventricular T wave. For this reason, most defibrillators have a synchronizing mechanism whereby discharge is triggered to occur at the time of the R or S wave. The synchronizing mechanism should be used during cardioversion for all arrhythmias with the exception of ventricular fibrillation. With ventricular fibrillation there will be no detectable R wave and thus, if the synchronizing mechanism is in operation, the defibrillator will not discharge. Before synchronized cardioversion, the operator should check that the synchronizing signal coincides with the onset of the QRS complex.

### Energy Levels

In general, low energy levels are used initially. If unsuccessful, further shocks can be given at increased levels. The initial energy setting depends on clinical circumstances. For example, atrial flutter usually responds to low energy shocks—25 Ws (Joules) would be an appropriate initial level. On the other hand, with ventricular fibrillation it is best to use a fairly high level—200 Ws initially. When digoxin toxicity is suspected, very low levels should be used, starting at 5–10 Ws. For other arrhythmias it is usual to start at 50 Ws and increase by increments of 50–100 Ws. Levels of 400 Ws should not be exceeded.

In children lower energy levels should be used, starting at 5–10 Ws.

### Complications

Complications are rare. Hypotension and heart failure are occasionally produced. Enzyme levels are elevated in some patients and may be due to either skeletal or cardiac muscle damage. Transient arrhythmias are sometimes induced by cardioversion but these are rarely a problem unless there is digoxin toxicity. In patients with the bradycardia–tachycardia syndrome a profound bradycardia may be caused by cardioversion. When this syndrome is suspected a temporary pacing wire should be inserted before cardioversion. Systemic embolism may occur when cardioversion is carried out for arrhythmias of supraventricular origin (*see below*).

Nitrate patches or paste should be removed from the chest to avoid the risk of explosion.

## Digoxin Toxicity

Cardioversion in the presence of digoxin toxicity can produce dangerous ventricular arrhythmias. For this reason cardioversion should be used as a last resort when there is digoxin toxicity and should be preceeded by lignocaine 75–100 mg. Because of the dangers of digoxin toxicity, it has become common practice to discontinue digoxin for 24–48 h prior to cardioversion in all cases. However, cardioversion in the presence of therapeutic levels of digoxin is safe. Cardioversion need not be postponed if one can be quite certain that digoxin toxicity is not present, i.e. the dose of digoxin is not excessive, renal function and plasma electrolytes are normal and there are no symptoms or ECG findings suggestive of digoxin toxicity.

## Anticoagulation

In patients with atrial fibrillation or flutter, thrombus may develop in the atria and be dislodged when sinus rhythm returns. For this rhythm anti-coagulation should be given before elective cardioversion when the cause of the arrhythmia is associated with a significant risk of systemic embolism, i.e. mitral valve disease, bradycardia–tachycardia syndrome and acute thyrotoxicosis. Oral anticoagulants should preferably be started 3 weeks before cardioversion and should be continued for 3 weeks afterwards.

# INDICATIONS

## Ventricular Fibrillation

Rarely, a praecordial blow will effect a return to sinus rhythm; otherwise, immediate cardioversion is indicated. The initial energy level should be 200 Ws. If unsuccessful the shock should be repeated at 300 or 400 Ws.

## Ventricular Tachycardia

Cardioversion should be carried out if the arrhythmia has caused shock or cardiac arrest, or if drug therapy has failed.

## Atrial Fibrillation

Cardioversion usually effects a return to sinus rhythm. The problem, however, is that atrial fibrillation returns in a high proportion of patients within a few months and often within hours of cardioversion. A long term successful result is more likely when cardiomegaly, left atrial enlargement and a long history of the arrhythmia are absent. Treatment with quinidine or disopyramide has been shown to increase modestly the chances of sinus rhythm being maintained.

### Atrial Flutter

This arrhythmia, which is often difficult to treat with drugs, responds to low energy shocks. The initial setting should be 25 Ws.

### Paroxysmal Supraventricular Tachycardia

Cardioversion is indicated on the occasions when other measures, such as vagal stimulation or intravenous verapamil, have failed.

## Main Points

1. The usual positions for the defibrillator paddles are the cardiac apex and to the right of the upper sternum. Firm pressure should be applied to the paddles when the DC shock is delivered.

2. With the exception of ventricular fibrillation, delivery of the shock should be synchronized to the R or S wave of the electrocardiogram.

3. Initial energy levels depend on the clinical circumstances: 25 Ws (Joules) for atrial flutter, 200 Ws for ventricular fibrillation, 50–100 Ws for most other arrhythmias.

4. Digoxin toxicity is a contraindication to cardioversion. Temporary transvenous pacing should be used to cover cardioversion if the brady-cardia-tachycardia syndrome is suspected.

5. In patients with atrial fibrillation or flutter due to conditions associated with a significant risk from systemic embolism, oral anti-coagulation for 3 weeks should precede cardioversion.

# Chapter 14

# Cardiac Arrest

Cardiac arrest is the cessation of an effective cardiac output as a result of a sudden circulatory or respiratory catastrophe. Patients dying from terminal and irreversible disease states will not benefit from and should not undergo the indignity of cardiopulmonary resuscitation.

## COMMON CAUSES

Acute myocardial infarction and severe coronary artery disease.
Anoxia, e.g. due to drowning, smoke inhalation, airways obstruction, respiratory depression.
Disease of the cardiac specialized conducting tissues.
Electrocution.
Iatrogenic, e.g. hypokalaemia or overdose of opiate, catecholamine.
Anaphylactic response to a drug or other allergens.

## DIAGNOSIS

Speed and efficiency in both the diagnosis and management of cardiac arrest are essential for a successful outcome.

Diagnosis of cardiac arrest is based on two signs: *Unconsciousness* and *Absent carotid or femoral artery pulsation.* Time should not be wasted in eliciting other signs of cardiac arrest, such as dilated pupils, apnoea, rigidity, pallor and absent heart sounds.

## MANAGEMENT

The management of cardiac arrest can be divided into three stages. First, establishment of an artificial circulation; secondly, restoration of spontaneous heart action; thirdly, after-care.

### 1. Artificial Circulation

Once the diagnosis of cardiac arrest has been made, immediate action should be taken.

First, a single blow should be given to the praecordium with the side of a clenched fist. Occasionally this will stop ventricular tachycardia or fibrillation. If unsuccessful, external cardiac massage and artificial respiration should be instituted immediately.

### External Cardiac Massage

Cardiac massage increases intrathoracic pressure and thereby propels blood into the arteries. Regurgitation into the venous system is prevented by valves at the superior thoracic inlet and, between chest compressions, the aortic valve remains competent, thus preventing blood flowing back into the heart.

The heel of one hand is placed over the sternum at the junction of its upper two-thirds and lower one-third and is covered by the other hand. Keeping the arms straight, the sternum should be depressed 3—4 cm at a rate of 60/min. Each compression should be sustained so that the time spent in compression is equal to that of relaxation.

It is rarely necessary to use all one's force in cardiac massage; a flail chest or visceral damage may result from over-enthusiastic massage.

The presence of arterial pulsation during cardiac massage is an encouraging sign although its absence does not necessarily mean that massage is ineffective.

### Artificial Respiration

If anoxia is the suspected cause of cardiac arrest, artificial respiration should be instituted before cardiac massage because there is little point in circulating hypoxic blood.

The patient's head should be tilted backwards, fully extending the neck. The lower jaw should be lifted forward so that it protrudes beyond the upper teeth. These manoeuvres will ensure that the tongue does not obstruct the airway. Mouth-to-mouth respiration should then be given by taking a deep breath and, after pinching the patient's nose, blowing forcefully into the patient's mouth, ensuring an airtight seal. The patient's chest should be seen to expand, otherwise respiration is inadequate. If chest expansion is not achieved after forceful blowing, the patient's pharynx should be examined to ensure that it is not obstructed by vomit or foreign material.

Twelve respirations per minute should be given. As respiration is given, cardiac massage should be interrupted. When there are two operators, the heart should be massaged five times and then the lungs ventilated once. Where there is only one operator, it is best to massage the heart ten times and then ventilate the lungs twice.

### Endotracheal Intubation

This is not necessary if spontaneous heart action can be restored quickly. If first attempts at restoration of heart action are unsuccessful, an endotracheal tube should be inserted. This has the advantages that it protects the airways from aspirated vomit and it allows pure oxygen to be given.

## 2. Restoration of Spontaneous Heart Action

Treatment depends on the heart rhythm. The paddles of a modern portable defibrillator also function as electrodes, enabling the heart rhythm to be quickly ascertained.

The ECG may reveal ventricular fibrillation, ventricular tachycardia, asystole or, very rarely, sinus rhythm. The latter may occur with a very large myocardial infarction, massive pulmonary embolism or cardiac tamponade, e.g. due to a ruptured left ventricle.

### Ventricular Fibrillation or Tachycardia

The patient should be immediately defibrillated. One of the major determinants of successful resuscitation is the delay before defibrillation. Though cardiac massage can maintain cerebral circulation for an appreciable time, there is little or no coronary artery blood flow during cardiac massage: the sooner spontaneous cardiac action can be restored, the better.

One paddle should be applied to the right of the upper sternum and the other to the cardiac apex. Electrode jelly or pads impregnated with electrode gel should be applied beneath the paddles. The defibrillator should be charged to 200 Ws. Everyone should be instructed to avoid contact with the patient, who is then defibrillated by pressing the button(s) on the defibrillator paddle(s). If 200 Ws is ineffective, repeat at 300 or 400 Ws. Trinitrin patches or paste applied to the chest should be removed before defibrillation as there is a small risk of explosion.

If there is ventricular tachycardia it is preferable, but not essential, to set the synchronizing mechanism so that the shock falls on the R wave rather than the T wave. If an unsynchronized shock causes ventricular fibrillation, a further shock must be given.

After reversion to sinus rhythm cardiac massage should be continued until there is a strong arterial pulse.

If the arrhythmia persists, cardiac massage and artificial respiration should be continued. Lignocaine (100 mg) should be given and acidosis should be corrected by 50 of 8·4 per cent sodium bicarbonate intravenously. Defibrillation should then be repeated at 400 Ws.

If defibrillation is again unsuccessful, further anti-arrhythmic therapy may help. A repeat bolus of lignocaine (75–100 mg) or mexiletine (100 mg) can be tried. Where the amplitude of the fibrillating waveform is small, 5–10 ml of 1 : 10 000 adrenaline should be used to coarsen 'fine' ventricular fibrillation. Further requirements for sodium bicarbonate can be estimated using the formula: ml required = body weight (kg) × duration of arrest (min) × 0·1.

It should be noted that if the defibrillator's synchronizing mechanism has been activated, the defibrillator will fail to discharge if there is ventricular fibrillation since no R waves will be detected. Though an obvious point, it is an occasional cause of failed defibrillation.

### Asystole

Resuscitation from asystole is often successful when the cause is anoxia or disease confined to the specialized conducting tissues. In the former case ventilation may be all that is required. In the latter case the mechanical stimulation of repeated praecordial blows or cardiac massage may initiate ventricular activation and maintain a satisfactory cardiac output. On the other hand, when asystole is due to extensive myocardial damage the prognosis is poor.

When ventilation and mechanical stimulation are ineffective, 10 ml of 10 per cent calcium chloride and 5 – 10 ml 1:10 000 adrenaline should be given. Acidosis should be reversed with sodium bicarbonate. Calcium chloride must not be given through the same line as sodium bicarbonate, without flushing the latter drug out, otherwise chalk will be formed. Further doses of adrenaline may be necessary – the asystolic heart can tolerate large doses of catecholamines. Defibrillation is useless in asystole.

Occasionally ventricular standstill may occur during atrial fibrillation and be confused with fine ventricular fibrillation.

### Sinus Rhythm

If cardiac arrest is thought to be due to cardiac tamponade, immediate aspiration of the pericardium or thoracotomy is indicated. Where pulmonary embolism is suspected, 15 000 units of heparin should be given intravenously. If facilities are to hand, emergency pulmonary embolectomy may be possible.

In patients with myocardial damage dissociation between electrical and mechanical activity can sometimes be reversed with intravenous calcium chloride and adrenaline.

### Administration of Drugs

Drugs given via a peripheral vein during cardiac arrest may not reach the heart. Instead, a line should be inserted into a central vein. The femoral vein is a good approach, since it is remote from the area of resuscitation. The external jugular vein is often distended during cardiac arrest, allowing easy cannulation. In some patients it may be necessary to cannulate the internal jugular or subclavian vein.

If a venous line cannot be established, adrenaline and lignocaine can be given via the intrapulmonary route. They should be diluted in 10 ml of saline and be given through a fine catheter, introduced via the endotracheal tube, deep into the lungs.

As a last resort intracardiac injection may be carried out. A long fine needle should be introduced either at the apex and advanced towards the right shoulder or through the fourth left intercoastal space, lateral to the sternum, until blood is aspirated.

## 3. After-care

The patient should be transferred to an intensive care unit. The heart rhythm should be monitored during transfer. If cardiac arrest was due to ventricular fibrillation or tachycardia, lignocaine or a second-line anti-arrhythmic agent should be given.

In patients who have been asystolic, unless there has been a readily reversible cause, e.g. anoxia, a temporary pacemaker should be inserted.

When there is impaired consciousness, intravenous dexamethasone (8 mg) and frusemide should be given to relieve cerebral oedema. Artificial ventilation may be necessary.

The blood acid-base state should be checked by analysis of arterial blood withdrawn from the femoral or radial artery. Acidosis should be reversed by giving 8·4 per cent sodium bicarbonate using the formula: ml required = body weight (kg) $\times$ 0·2 $\times$ base deficit.

## Main Points

1. Loss of consciousness plus absence of pulsation in a large artery are the only signs required for a diagnosis of cardiac arrest.

2. Cardiac massage is often poorly done. Precise positioning of the hands, at the junction of the upper two-thirds and lower one-third of the sternum, is essential. (Not infrequently 'cardiac massage' is applied to the epigastrium.) The operator's arms should be kept straight by 'locking the elbows', with the shoulders positioned directly over the hands. The chest should be compressed 60 times per minute, the duration of each compression should be sustained and equal to the relaxation phase.

3. Maintenance of a clear airway by full extension of the neck is essential for effective mouth-to-mouth resuscitation.

4. If there is ventricular fibrillation, the sooner defibrillation is carried out the more likely is a successful outcome. Initially, 200 J (Ws) should be used, the two paddles being positioned at the cardiac apex and to the right of the upper sternum. To avoid one common cause of delay, it is important one is familiar with the controls of the defibrillator(s) that one is likely to use.

# Chapter 15

# Temporary Cardiac Pacing

## INDICATIONS

### Stokes—Adams Attacks

A temporary pacemaker should be inserted in patients with syncope or near-syncope whether caused by impaired sinus node function or AV conduction. Unless the arrhythmia can be attributed to an acute event, e.g. myocardial infarction or digoxin toxicity, implantation of a permanent pacemaker should then be considered.

In patients with a history of recent syncope who are being referred to a cardiac centre for permanent pacing, a temporary pacemaker should be inserted before transfer because syncope may occur during transit with possibly irreversible consequences. This may not be essential, however, when symptoms are very infrequent and the heart rate is satisfactory.

### Heart Block in Acute Myocardial Infarction

In inferior infarction pacing is only necessary in the minority of cases where second or third degree AV block causes ventricular standstill, a very low ventricular rate (<40/min), ventricular arrhythmias, heart failure, hypotension or other signs of a low cardiac output (*see* Chapter 11).

In anterior infarction a temporary pacemaker should be inserted in all cases of second and third degree AV block because of the high likelihood of a profound bradycardia or asystole. In addition, pacing is indicated when there is evidence of extensive bundle branch damage (i.e. alternating right and left bundle branch block, or right bundle branch block plus left anterior or posterior fascicular block) because of the high risk that complete AV block will develop (*see* Chapter 11).

Symptomatic sinus arrest or junctional bradycardia, unresponsive to atropine, may also necessitate pacing.

### General Anaesthesia

Patients with second and third degree AV block should have a pacemaker to cover the operative period.

In the absence of a history of syncope, the risk of AV block developing during anaesthesia in a patient with evidence of bilateral bundle branch disease is very low and pacing is not essential.

## Tachycardias

Pacing is a useful method for terminating paroxysmal supraventricular tachycardia, atrial flutter and ventricular tachycardia. The most common methods are to pace either at rates faster (overdrive) or considerably slower (underdrive) than that of the tachycardia with the aim of suppressing automaticity of an ectopic focus or interrupting a circus movement mechanism.

In the bradycardia–tachycardia syndrome cardioversion may lead to a profound bradycardia. Temporary pacing is indicated to cover cardioversion in patients with a tachycardia of supraventricular origin in whom the sick sinus syndrome is suspected.

## METHODS

Temporary ventricular pacing is usually carried out by introducing a transvenous pacing electrode under local anaesthesia into a systemic vein and advancing it, with the aid of X-ray screening, to the right ventricle. The electrode is connected to an external battery-powered pulse generator. During insertion the heart rhythm must be monitored and equipment for resuscitation should be available.

Transthoracic rather than transvenous electrodes are used for temporary pacing in open heart surgery and they can also be used percutaneously in an emergency when screening facilities are not available.

### Subclavian Vein Puncture

The subclavian vein is the most suitable route of access to the venous system. The vein runs behind the medial third of the clavicle and can be punctured using either supraclavicular or infraclavicular approaches. Only the latter will be described.

The patient should be laid flat or, if possible, in a slight head-down position. A needle is introduced, through a ½-cm skin incision, just below the inferior border of the clavicle, slightly medial to the mid-clavicular point, and is directed towards the sternoclavicular joint so that it passes immediately behind the posterior surface of the clavicle. When first advancing the needle it is advisable to locate the clavicle with the needle in order to avoid going in too deeply, with consequent risk of pneumothorax or subclavian artery puncture.

As the needle punctures the vein, venous blood will be easily aspirated. If there is only a trickle of blood it is unlikely that the needle tip is in the subclavian vein.

Cannulation of the vein is best achieved by introducing a guide wire through the needle into the vein. A guide wire with a flexible J-shaped tip is much easier to advance around the junction between the subclavian vein and superior vena cava, which can often be quite an acute bend. The needle is then withdrawn and a sheath within which there is a vessel dilator is passed over the wire into the vein. The guide wire and dilator are then removed, and the pacing lead is passed through the sheath. It is important to ensure before vein puncture that the lead will easily pass through the sheath.

The main advantages of subclavian vein puncture are that it is quick and infection and electrode displacement are unusual. Possible complications, which are rare in experienced hands, are pneumothorax, haemothorax, subclavian artery puncture and air embolism.

### Antecubital Vein Cut-down

It is important to select a medially situated vein. It is unusual to be able to negotiate an electrode into the superior vena cava from a lateral vein.

The disadvantages of this method are that electrode stability is poor, even when the patient's arm is strapped to his side, and infection and phlebitis are not uncommon.

### Femoral Vein Puncture

This method is very easy and quick, provided that pulsation of the laterally adjacent femoral artery is easily palpable. However, it should be reserved for short term emergency purposes because electrode stability is poor and there is a risk of venous thrombosis. Pressure on the abdomen causes distension of the femoral vein and makes venepuncture easier.

### Positioning of the Electrode

If there is resistance to the introduction of the electrode into the vein, it is probable that the lumen has not been entered. Once in the venous system, it should be possible to advance the electrode without any resistance. If an obstruction is encountered, the electrode should be withdrawn slightly, rotated and then advanced again. Nothing will be achieved by forcing the electrode.

Once the electrode has reached the right atrium, a loop should be formed by impinging the electrode tip on the atrial wall (*Fig.* 15.1A) and then advancing the electrode a little further (*Fig.* 15.1B). By twisting the electrode, the loop is then rotated so that the electrode tip lies near the tricuspid valve (*Fig.* 15.1C). Slight withdrawal of the electrode will allow the tip to 'flick' through the valve into the right ventricle.

Ventricular ectopic beats are usually provoked as the valve is crossed. If these do not occur it is possible that the coronary sinus rather than the right ventricle has been entered. An electrode lying in the coronary sinus assumes a characteristic shape (*Fig.* 15.1F). (A lateral view will show that

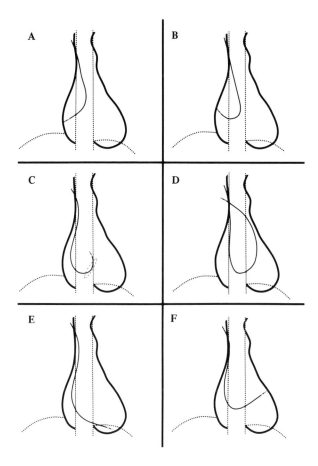

*Fig.* 15.1. Diagrams illustrating insertion of a transvenous pacing lead. A loop is formed in the right atrium (A and B). The loop is positioned near the tricuspid valve, indicated by the oval of dashes (C). Entry into the right ventricle can be confirmed by passing the wire into the pulmonary artery (D). The pacing lead is then positioned in the apex of the right ventricle (E). F, The characteristic appearance of a pacing lead in the coronary sinus.

the electrode is pointing posteriorly whereas an electrode in the right ventricular apex points anteriorly.) It can be confirmed that the right ventricle has been entered by advancing the electrode into the pulmonary artery (*Fig.* 15.1D).

Once in the right ventricle, the electrode tip is positioned in or near the apex of the ventricle by a process of advancement, withdrawal and rotation (*Fig.* 15.1E).

Difficulty with electrode manipulation can be due to poor technique. Another cause is that re-useable pacing electrodes lose their stiffness after repeated use and should not be employed more than six times. If positioning proves difficult, it is well worth trying a new electrode.

## Pacing

When a stable electrode position in or near the right ventricular apex has been achieved, the distal and proximal poles of the electrode should be connected to the pacemaker cathode (−) and anode (+), respectively. If the poles are connected the other way round, the stimulation threshold will be substantially higher. The pacing threshold, which is the minimum voltage necessary for pacing stimuli to capture the ventricles consistently, should then be measured (*Fig.* 15.2). It should be less than 1·0 volt (assuming that the temporary pacemaker delivers impulses whose duration is 2 ms. Some temporary pacemakers allow the pulse width to be adjustable: shorter pulse widths will lead to a higher threshold and are virtually never indicated for temporary pacing). If not, the electrode should, if possible, be repositioned.

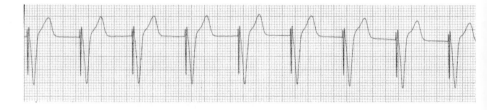

*Fig.* 15.2. Ventricular pacing (lead II). Each pacing stimulus is followed by a ventricular complex. An electrode positioned in the apex of the right ventricle will produce left axis deviation of the paced beats.

Sometimes, particularly in an emergency, a pacing threshold or electrode position which is less than optimal has to be accepted. Occasionally a patient may become dependent on the pacemaker, making adjustment of the electrode position hazardous. In these circumstances it may be necessary to insert a second pacing electrode (e.g. via the femoral vein) to cover the period of repositioning.

The stability of the pacing lead should be tested by ensuring that there is consistent pacing during coughing and deep inspiration. During the latter manoeuvre, if there is the correct amount of slack in the lead, there will be a slight curve in its right atrial portion (*Fig.* 15.1E). It is essential for lead stability that the electrode be securely sutured to the skin at its point of entry.

The pacing threshold usually rises to 2–3 V during the first few days after electrode insertion. The threshold should be checked daily and the voltage set at twice the measured threshold. Battery function and electrical connections should also be checked daily.

## Pacing Complications

Causes of failure to pace (*Fig.* 15.3) include electrode displacement, myocardial perforation, exit block and a break in either the electrical connections or the pacing electrode.

Electrode displacement may cause intermittent or complete failure to pace. The electrode may fall back into the right atrial cavity and lead to atrial rather than ventricular pacing (*Fig.* 15.4).

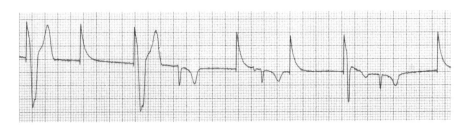

*Fig.* 15.3. Intermittent failure to pace (lead II). Only the first and third pacing stimuli capture the ventricles.

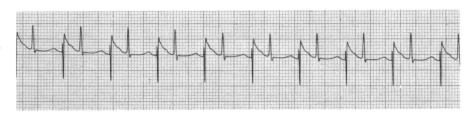

*Fig.* 15.4. Atrial pacing. At the time of this recording, AV function was satisfactory so each pacing stimulus was followed by a narrow QRS complex after a PR interval of 0·22 s.

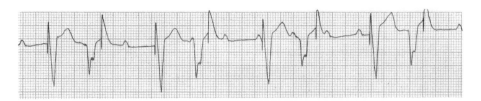

*Fig.* 15.5. Failure to sense in a demand ventricular pacemaker. The first, third, fifth and seventh pacing stimuli capture the ventricles. The second, fourth, sixth and eighth stimuli fall on the T waves of spontaneous ventricular beats.

Occasionally the electrode tip may perforate the thin right ventricular myocardium. This is more common with disposable electrodes, which tend to be stiffer than re-useable ones. Failure to pace, diaphragmatic stimulation, pericardial friction rub and pericardial pain may result. Cardiac tamponade is extremely rare.

Sometimes pacing failure occurs without obvious electrode tip displacement or other cause. In these cases failure is attributed to 'exit block', the cause of which is thought to be excessive tissue reaction at the junction between electrode tip and endocardium.

A break in the electrical connections or in the electrode itself can be the cause of intermittent or complete pacing failure. In contrast to exit block, no pacing stimuli will appear on the ECG. Another occasional cause of pacing failure associated with absent pacing stimuli is external inhibition of a demand pacemaker usually resulting from electromagnetic waves being emitted from electrical equipment. This problem can be quickly solved by changing the pacemaker to fixed rate mode.

Pacemakers are most often used in the 'demand' mode, whereby the pacemaker senses spontaneous ventricular activity and only discharges a stimulus if a spontaneous beat has not occurred within a pre-set period. In some patients, particularly those with myocardial infarction, the signal generated by spontaneous activity may be too small for the pacemaker to sense. As a result, the pacemaker will function in a 'fixed rate' mode and pacing stimuli will be discharged at inappropriate times, and may fall on the T wave of a spontaneous beat (*Fig.* 15.5). This is particularly undesirable in acute myocardial infarction because of the risk of precipitating ventricular fibrillation.

As an alternative to electrode repositioning, unipolar pacing can be adopted. In contrast to bipolar pacing, the anode is remote from the electrode tip. The signal generated by spontaneous activity sensed between two poles separated by a large distance is much greater. Unipolar pacing can be achieved by disconnecting the pacemaker connection to the proximal pole of the pacing electrode and connecting it to a needle inserted beneath the skin in a convenient position which functions as the remote pole.

The site of entry of a transvenous pacing electrode can become infected: sometimes bacteraemia results. Infection will not clear up without removal of the pacing electrode. If necessary, a new pacing electrode will have to be inserted at a different site.

## AV Sequential Pacing

Ventricular pacing results in dissociation between atrial and ventricular activity. When ventricular systole is not immediately preceded by atrial systole, cardiac output falls by up to one-third. It is possible to pace both the atria and ventricles sequentially so that the normal sequence of cardiac chamber activation can be maintained (*Fig.* 15.6). In patients with

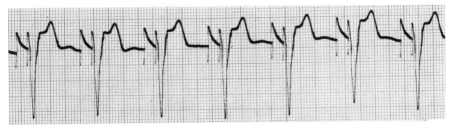

*Fig.* 15.6. AV sequential pacing. Pacing stimuli precede both atrial and ventricular complexes.

a low cardiac output, AV sequential pacing can produce an important improvement in cardiac function.

Usually, AV sequential pacing is achieved by passing two leads to the heart: one to the atria and one to the ventricles. The best method of ensuring that an atrial lead is not displaced is to use one with a pre-formed J-shaped terminal portion. A lead of this type can easily be positioned in the right atrial appendage (*see* Chapter 16). Recently, 'single-pass' leads with a distal electrode for ventricular pacing and a proximal pole for atrial pacing have been introduced for AV sequential pacing.

## Main Points

**1.** Indications for temporary transvenous pacing include bifascicular, second and third degree AV block due to acute anterior infarction; 'complicated' second and third degree AV block due to acute inferior infarction; and recent syncope or near-syncope due to chronic disease of the sinus node or AV junction while awaiting implantation of a long term pacemaker.

**2.** Subclavian vein puncture is usually the best method of venous access for temporary pacing.

**3.** The pacemaker stimulation threshold, battery function and electrical connections should be checked daily.

**4.** AV sequential pacing improves cardiac output as compared with ventricular pacing and should be considered in those patients whose haemodynamic status is not satisfactory with ventricular pacing.

# Chapter 16

# Long Term Cardiac Pacing

The first pacemaker was implanted in 1958. Since then, progress in pacemaker technology and an increasing awareness of the benefits of pacing have led to a steady rise each year in the number of patients receiving pacemakers. In the United Kingdom, approximately 115 per million of the population receive a pacemaker each year. In most European countries, the implantation rate is more than twice as high and in America the rate is four times that of the UK.

Patients of all ages, from the newborn to those over 100 years, have been paced. The average age at first implantation is 68 years.

## INDICATIONS

### Complete AV Block

The most common indication for pacemaker implantation is prevention of syncope or near-syncope.

Though some patients may experience Stokes—Adams attacks for many years without permanent sequelae, in general the prognosis for patients with Stokes—Adams attacks is poor; 1-year survival rates as low as 50 per cent have been reported. After pacemaker implantation, the prognosis is much improved. In those without ischaemic heart disease or myocardial failure, the survival rate closely approaches that of the general population.

In most patients a single episode of syncope or near-syncope is sufficient to warrant a pacemaker. As the next Stokes—Adams attack may be fatal or cause injury, delay in referral should be minimal.

In the very elderly and those with other major illnesses, improvement in prognosis may not be an important consideration. Even in these patients, however, pacing should be considered because by preventing blackouts, confidence, independence and mobility may be preserved and serious injury, which may lead to greater demands on medical resources than pacemaker implantation, may be avoided.

Heart block may cause a reduction in cardiac output leading to dyspnoea on effort, tiredness and heart failure. These symptoms often, but not invariably, improve with pacing.

There is evidence to suggest that prognosis in asymptomatic heart block is improved by pacing. Certainly, pacing should be considered in younger patients.

## First and Second Degree AV Block

Patients with syncope sometimes present with first or second degree AV block. In those with Mobitz type II block, provided that the symptoms are consistent with Stokes–Adams attacks, it can be assumed that intermittent complete AV block is responsible for the symptoms and a pacemaker should be inserted.

In patients with first degree or Wenkebach block, intermittent complete block may well be responsible for the symptoms, but a higher degree of AV block should, if possible, be documented before pacemaker implantation, e.g. by ambulatory ECG monitoring.

## Bundle Branch Blocks

Frequently patients with syncope present with evidence of bundle branch or bifascicular block. As with Mobitz type II AV block, it is likely that intermittent deterioration in infranodal conduction causes complete AV block and consequent syncope.

In patients with bifascicular block (complete left bundle branch block or left anterior or posterior fascicular block plus right bundle branch block) pacemaker implantation is indicated provided that symptoms are consistent with Stokes–Adams attacks. In those patients with atypical symptoms and in those with isolated right bundle branch block, which is a common finding in otherwise normal hearts, further investigations such as ambulatory ECG monitoring or perhaps intracardiac electrophysiological testing (see Chapter 19) are necessary.

In asymptomatic patients with bifascicular block, the chances of progression to complete AV block, with consequent risk of syncope or sudden death, is in the order of a few per cent each year. However, because the timing of these events cannot be predicted and because the major determinant of prognosis in these patients is the presence of coronary artery or myocardial disease, prophylactic pacing is not indicated.

## Sick Sinus Syndrome

Over a quarter of pacemakers currently implanted are for treatment of the sick sinus syndrome. Pacemaker implantation is indicated in patients who experience syncope or near-syncope. In addition, patients with brady-cardia–tachycardia syndrome may require pacemaker implantation to cover anti-arrhythmic therapy (see Chapter 10).

The prognosis for sick sinus syndrome is quite good and is better than for AV block. Prophylactic pacing is therefore not necessary in asymptomatic patients for the purpose of improving prognosis. However, pacing should still be considered in asymptomatic patients who are found to have long pauses in cardiac activity since they are at risk from injury if syncope does occur. This is a particularly important consideration in car drivers.

### Syncope with a Normal ECG

This is a common problem. Patients with symptoms due to sick sinus syndrome often have a normal routine ECG. Sometimes patients with paroxysmal complete AV block also have a normal routine ECG. Unless there are exceptional circumstances, abnormalities in conduction should be documented by ambulatory ECG monitoring (several recordings may be necessary) or, occasionally, by intracardiac electrophysiological testing before a pacemaker is inserted.

### Paroxysmal Tachycardia

In patients with paroxysmal tachycardias unresponsive to anti-arrhythmic therapy, long term cardiac pacing may be indicated (*see* Chapters 5, 6, 15).

### Heart Block in Myocardial Infarction

As discussed in Chapter 11, permanent AV block after inferior infarction is extremely unusual and long term pacing is thus rarely required.

In complete AV block complicating anterior infarction, block sometimes persists and necessitates long term pacing. When AV conduction recovers, there is often residual bifascicular block. In these patients complete AV block may recur after discharge from hospital and may result in sudden death. As discussed in Chapter 11, there is no conclusive evidence to show that long term pacing will improve the prognosis. Many of these patients have had extensive myocardial damage and, as a result, are at risk from ventricular fibrillation and heart failure, whether or not they are paced. In some patients, however, clinical and biochemical evidence suggests that myocardial infarction might not be extensive. In these patients permanent pacing may be advantageous.

## PACING MODES

All pacing systems consist of a pulse generator connected to an electrode or electrodes in contact with an endocardial or epicardial surface.

### Fixed Rate and Demand Pacing Systems

The simplest mode of pacing is fixed rate (or asynchronous) pacing. Fixed rate pacing was widely used in the early years of pacing but has now been largely superseded by demand systems. A fixed rate pacemaker discharges regularly, usually at a rate of 70/min, irrespective of spontaneous cardiac activity (*Fig.* 16.1). As a result, the paced rhythm may compete with a spontaneous rhythm and cause unpleasant, irregular palpitation (*Fig.* 16.2). In the case of ventricular pacing, stimuli will coincide at times with the T waves of spontaneous beats and may possibly induce ventricular fibrillation. In practice, ventricular fibrillation is a rare event except in acute myocardial infarction, from which pacemaker patients are not immune. In fixed rate atrial pacing stimuli may fall during the atrial recovery period and induce atrial fibrillation.

Demand pacemakers can be reset by spontaneous cardiac activity, which is sensed through the stimulating electrode, and thus avoid competition

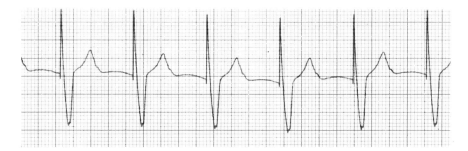

*Fig.* 16.1   Fixed rate ventricular pacing at 71 beats/min.

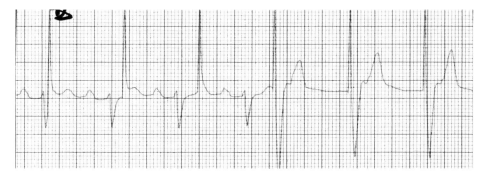

*Fig.* 16.2. Fixed rate ventricular pacing in a patient with first degree AV block. The first three stimuli fall during the refractory period and are ineffective. The fourth causes a premature contraction.

between paced and spontaneous rhythms. If there is no spontaneous activity, the pacemaker functions as though it were a fixed rate pacemaker.

Most demand systems are of the 'inhibited' type. The pacemaker is inhibited by intrinsic cardiac activity and will only discharge if a spon-

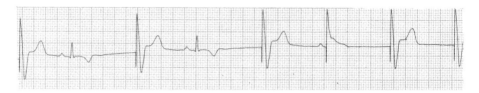

*Fig.* 16.3. Demand ventricular pacemaker. The pacemaker is inhibited by the sinus beats (second and fourth complexes). The sixth complex is a fusion beat. A P wave can be seen to precede the pacing stimulus. By chance, a sinus impulse has arisen at the instant when the pacemaker was set to discharge and the ventricles have been activated by both sinus impulse and pacemaker. Fusion beats should not be confused with failure to pace.

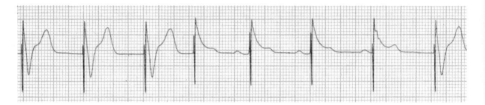

*Fig.* 16.4. Ventricular triggered pacemaker. After the first three paced beats there is sinus rhythm. A pacing stimulus is discharged immediately after the onset of the QRS complex in these beats.

taneous beat has not occurred within a pre-set period, which is in the order of 0·8–1·0 s (*Fig.* 16.3).

A less commonly used system is the 'triggered' type. The pacemaker discharges continuously but any spontaneous beats re-set the pacemaker so that stimuli fall immediately after ventricular activation, during the myocardial refractory period, and are therefore ineffective (*Fig.* 16.4).

## Atrial Demand Pacing

This is the ideal pacing mode for patients with the sick sinus syndrome (*Fig.* 16.5). First, by stimulating the atria, it maintains the normal sequence of cardiac chamber activation, loss of which can reduce the cardiac output at rest by up to one-third. Secondly, in patients with the bradycardia-tachycardia syndrome, atrial pacing ensures regular atrial systole and hence may reduce the risk of systemic embolism due to atrial statis and may prevent tachyarrhythmias of supraventricular origin when these arise as escape rhythms during bradycardia.

Clearly, atrial pacing is inappropriate in patients with impaired AV conduction. Some patients with sick sinus syndrome also have disease of the AV junction. If this is apparent from the electrocardiogram or if atrial pacing at 120 beats/min causes second or third degree AV block, an atrial pacemaker is unsuitable and AV sequential or ventricular pacing should be

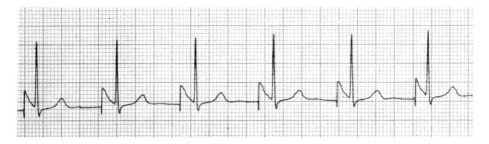

*Fig.* 16.5. Atrial pacing.

considered. Several studies have shown that if AV conduction is satisfactory at the time of atrial pacemaker implantation, then there is only a small chance of deterioration in conduction (which would necessitate a change of pacing system) over the ensuing years.

Atrial pacing is contraindicated if there is atrial fibrillation, flutter or tachycardia unless these rhythm disturbances arise during atrial bradycardia, in which case atrial pacing may well prevent them.

## Ventricular Demand Pacing

This is the simplest and most widely used form of pacing (*see Fig.* 16.1). Many patients benefit from this pacing mode but it has two disadvantages, both of which can lead to symptoms due to an inadequate cardiac output.

### Pacemaker Syndrome

Ventricular pacing prevents the normal sequence of cardiac chamber activation. Usually atrial activity becomes dissociated from ventricular activity but in some patients, particularly those with sick sinus syndrome or lower degrees of AV block, the AV junction will transmit the ventricular stimulus back to the atria, resulting in retrograde atrial activation (*Fig.* 16.6). This is haemodynamically worse than AV dissociation.

When normal AV synchrony is lost, atrial contraction may occur against closed mitral and tricuspid valves. As a consequence, atrial pressure will rise and impede venous return so that during the next diastolic period the ventricle will be underfilled with a resultant reduction in stroke volume. Loss of properly timed atrial systole results in a reduction of resting cardiac output by up to 30 per cent and hence a fall in blood pressure (*Fig.* 16.7), which, in spite of reflex vasoconstriction, may cause symptomatic hypotension – dizziness, near-syncope and syncope can occur. Hypotension is most severe during the first few seconds of ventricular pacing, before compensatory mechanisms can come into play, so ventricular pacing is particularly unsuitable for patients who are usually in sinus rhythm but who often develop bradycardia at a rate less than the demand rate of the ventricular pacemaker.

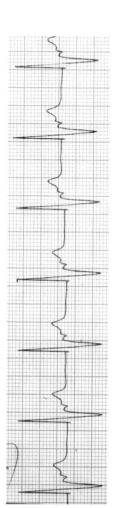

*Fig.* 16.6.   Ventricular pacing with retrograde atrial activation (lead II). Each ventricular complex is followed by a P wave.

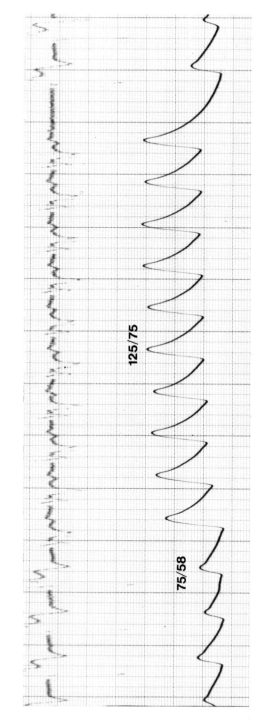

*Fig.* 16.7.   Pacemaker syndrome. Effect of ventricular pacing on arterial pressure. There was symptomatic hypotension during right ventricular pacing. After the first four paced beats the pacemaker is inhibited by an external pacemaker (chest wall stimulation), allowing sinus rhythm to resume control of the heart with consequent increase in pressure. The arterial pressure falls during the last two beats, when ventricular pacing restarts.

## Lack of Chronotropic Response to Exercise

The rate of impulse discharge from a ventricular demand pacemaker does not increase during exercise. As discussed below, this lack of a chronotropic response can markedly limit a patient's exercise tolerance.

Many patients who receive benefit from ventricular demand pacemakers would be further improved by more sophisticated pacing systems that maintain the normal sequence of cardiac chamber activation and/or provide a chronotropic response to exercise. As pacing technology improves and the awareness of the benefits of 'physiological pacing' increase, it is likely that the ventricular demand mode will be used less often. However, unequivocal indications for ventricular demand pacing include bradycardia associated with persistent atrial fibrillation, complete heart block in patients who are limited by impaired cerebral or locomotor function, and patients with infrequent bradycardia in whom the pacemaker is mainly on 'standby'.

### AV Sequential Pacing

In this pacing mode, the atria are stimulated first, and after an interval which approximates to that of the normal PR interval, the ventricles are stimulated (*Fig.* 16.8). Both atrial and ventricular pacing leads are required. This system maintains the normal sequence of cardiac chamber activation but does not provide a chronotropic response to exercise.

The main indication is for the sick sinus syndrome associated with impaired AV conduction. The pacemaker functions in the demand mode: it is inhibited by spontaneous ventricular activity.

### Atrial Synchronized Ventricular Pacing

This system both maintains normal AV synchrony and causes the ventricular stimulation rate to increase in response to the rate of sinus node discharge. Like AV sequential pacing, both atrial and ventricular electrodes are required. Activity sensed by the atrial electrode triggers ventricular stimulation via the ventricular electrode after a delay similar

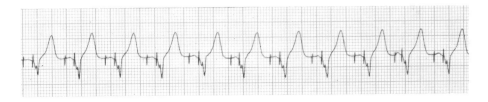

*Fig.* 16.8. AV sequential pacing. Pacing stimuli precede both atrial and ventricular complexes.

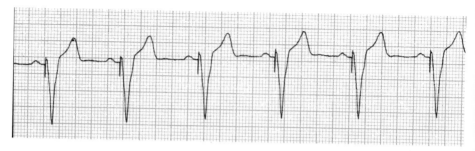

*Fig*. 16.9. Atrial synchronized pacing. Each P wave is followed by a paced ventricular beat.

to the normal PR interval (*Fig*. 16.9). The pacemaker is not inhibited by ventricular ectopic beats. There is an upper limit to the ventricular response so that the ventricles are protected should atrial fibrillation or flutter develop.

The main indication for atrial synchronized ventricular pacing is in patients with second or third degree AV block who do not have atrial tachyarrhythmias or impaired sinus node function.

Atrial synchronized ventricular pacing usually improves exercise tolerance as compared with ventricular demand pacing — in part because it maintains AV synchrony but mainly because it facilitates a chronotropic response to exercise.

Several double-blind studies have been conducted to compare exercise tolerance during ventricular and atrial synchronized pacing. These have demonstrated that overall exercise tolerance is improved by about one-third to a half by the latter mode. However, the degree of benefit varies from patient to patient. In some the improvement is dramatic whereas in others it is minimal. Unfortunately, it is impossible to predict who is not going to benefit substantially from this pacing mode.

### The 'Universal Pacemaker'

This pacemaker combines the benefits of AV sequential and atrial synchronized ventricular pacing. It senses activity both in the atrium and ventricle. If there is sinus bradycardia, it functions as an atrial demand pacemaker. If there is impaired AV conduction, ventricular pacing is triggered by either spontaneous P waves or by atrial pacing. When sinus node function is normal, it acts in the atrial synchronized mode thus providing a chronotropic response to exercise. The pacemaker is inhibited by both atrial and ventricular ectopic beats (*Fig*. 16.10).

This pacing mode has largely superseded use of pacemakers that can only function as AV sequential or atrial synchronized systems. Like other systems involving the use of an atrial lead, the 'universal' pacemaker is contraindicated if there are persistent or frequent atrial tachyarrhythmias.

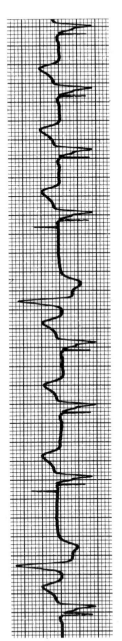

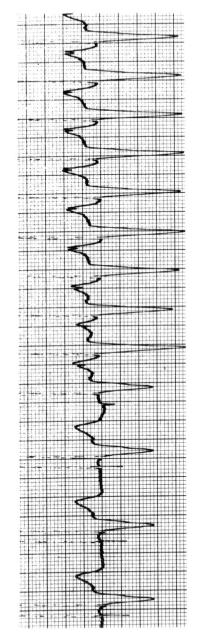

*Fig.* 16.10. Universal (DDD) pacing. Spontaneous P waves can be seen to trigger ventricular stimulation. After the first and fifth paced beats there are ventricular ectopic beats which inhibit the pacemaker. There is sinus node depression following the extrasytoles to which the pacemaker responds by pacing the atria as well as the ventricles.

*Fig.* 16.11. Pacemaker-mediated tachycardia develops after four cycles of AV sequential pacing.

'Universal' pacing can cause an important complication: pacemaker mediated tachycardia (*Fig.* 16.11). This can occur if the AV junction is capable of conducting ventricular stimuli back to the atria and does so at a relatively slow speed. If retrograde atrial activation is sensed through the atrial lead, the pacemaker will automatically trigger ventricular stimulation which will again result in retrograde atrial activation and hence a pacemaker-mediated tachycardia similar in mechanism to AV re-entrant tachycardia (*see* Chapter 6). This problem can usually be solved by prolonging the refractory period of the atrial sensing circuit so that retrograde atrial stimuli arrive at the atrial lead while the atrial sensing circuit is not functioning. Pacemakers are being developed which can recognize the onset of and therefore interrupt pacemaker-mediated tachycardia.

## 'Rate Responsive' Pacing

There are three disadvantages to the use of atrial synchronized ventricular pacing for the provision of a chronotropic response to exercise: two pacing leads are required; pacemaker-mediated tachycardia may occur; and the pacing mode relies on normal or near-normal sinus node function.

Several alternative pacing systems have been developed whose discharge rate can vary according to a sensed parameter which alters with exercise, e.g. respiration, blood temperature, blood pH or the intracardiac equivalent of the QT interval (which shortens with increased sympathetic nervous system activity). These systems do not require an atrial lead and do not therefore have the disadvantages of atrial synchronized pacing. They do not, of course, maintain AV synchrony. However, as mentioned above, AV synchrony is not nearly as important as a chronotropic response in providing a good exercise tolerance. These rate-responsive systems are still in their infancy. They only require one pacing lead and can be used in spite of atrial fibrillation. They will, however, not be suitable for patients who experience the pacemaker syndrome.

## Pacing System Code

A five-character code is now widely used to describe the various different types of pacing system. The first character indicates the chamber or chambers paced, the second indicates the chamber or chambers whose activity is sensed and the third indicates how the pacemaker responds to the sensed information. The fourth and fifth characters are optional: the fourth indicates whether the pacemaker is programmable and the fifth whether it has anti-tachycardia functions. As pacing gets more sophisticated it is likely that the code will have to be modified, but it is certain that it will not get any simpler (Table 16.1). (In the code, D is an abbreviation for double, indicating that both atria and ventricles are involved or, in the case of the third character, that the pacemaker responds both in triggered and inhibited modes.)

*Table* 16.1. Five-character pacemaker code

| Position | I | II | III | IV | V |
|---|---|---|---|---|---|
| *Category* | Chamber(s) paced | Chamber(s) sensed | Mode of response(s) | Programmable functions | Special tachyarrhythmia functions |
| *Letters used* | V–Ventricle | V–Ventricle | T–Triggered | P–Programmable (rate and/or output) | B–Bursts |
| | A–Atrium | A–Atrium | I–Inhibited | M–Multiprogrammable | N–Normal rate completion |
| | D–Double | D–Double | D–Double O–None | | S–Scanning |
| | | O–None | R–Reverse | O–None | E–External |

For example, a ventricular demand pacemaker stimulates the ventricles and is inhibited by spontaneous ventricular activity: the appropriate code is therefore VVI. Similarly, an atrial demand pacemaker is represented by AAI. An atrial synchronized ventricular pacemaker is triggered by sensed atrial activity and is therefore represented by VAT. DVI indicates that both atria and ventricles are paced and that the pacemaker is inhibited by activity sensed from the ventricles, i.e. an AV sequential pacemaker. A 'universal' pacemaker can stimulate both the atria and ventricles, it can be both inhibited by spontaneous activity sensed from either set of chambers and can be triggered by sensed atrial activity, and is therefore represented by DDD.

## PACEMAKER GENERATORS

### Power Sources

A number of power sources have been used in pacemaker generators, including mercury–zinc cells, rechargeable nickel–cadmium, lithium iodide and other lithium salt cells and nuclear energy. Now lithium batteries are used almost exclusively; they have replaced the other widely used power source, the mercury–zinc cell, whose lifetime was limited to 3–4 years. Lithium-powered pacemakers have a minimum lifetime of 4 years and some have an anticipated life expectancy in excess of 15 years.

Over the years, the size of pacemaker generators has been reduced. The modern pacemaker is compact and unobtrusive, being about 0·8 cm thick and having a maximum diameter of about 5 cm.

### Programmable Pacemakers

A programmable pacemaker can be non-invasively adjusted in one or more of its functions by an external programmer which emits electromagnetic coded signals. Programmable pacemakers allow 'fine tuning' of various

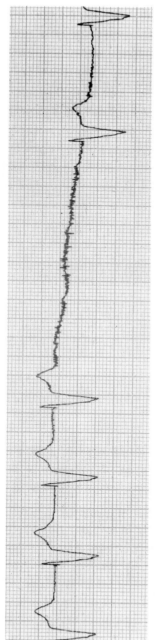

*Fig.* 16.12. Electromyographic inhibition of a ventricular demand pacemaker. Each time the patient lifted his arm, he felt dizzy. Corrected by programming to VVT.

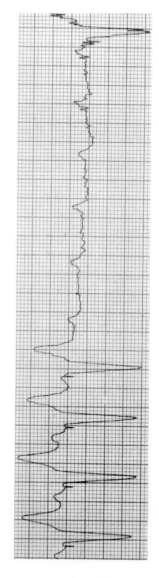

*Fig.* 16.13. Electromyographic inhibition of a universal (DDD) pacemaker. Activities such as washing hands caused near-syncope. Corrected by decreasing pacemaker sensitivity.

parameters to achieve optimal pacing for a given clinical situation (which may change from time to time) and also permit diagnosis and treatment of a variety of pacemaker complications that would otherwise necessitate re-operation. Many would argue that non-programmable pacemakers should no longer be used. Not only can pacemakers be externally programmed but some can be interrogated as to a wide variety of information about pacemaker and cardiac activity.

Simple programmable pacemakers can be adjusted for stimulation rate and output. With 'multi-programmable' pacemakers several other parameters can be non-invasively adjusted: pacemaker sensitivity, mode (e.g. inhibited, fixed rate, triggered), refractory period duration (the period during which sensing circuits are inactive), and in the case of dual chamber pacemakers, the duration of AV delay.

A few examples of the use of pacemaker programmability are given below:

1. *Battery life*. The stimulation threshold is usually a lot lower than the pacemaker's output. Threshold can be measured by progressive reduction in output until there is failure to capture. By reducing output to twice or thrice the threshold value, battery life can be conserved.

2. *Pacemaker syndrome*. In patients who are mainly in sinus rhythm, the standby rate of a demand pacemaker can be reduced (e.g. to 50 or 60/min) to avoid competition with normal sinus rhythm and reduce problems due to the pacemaker syndrome.

3. *Ventricular arrhythmias*. Sometimes, an increase in pacing rate will suppress arrhythmias.

4. *Extracardiac stimulation*. Pacemakers occasionally stimulate underlying muscle or the diaphragm. Reduction of output will usually prevent extracardiac stimulation.

5. *Electromyographic (EMG) inhibition*. Not infrequently, electrical activity from the pectoral muscle in contact with the pacemaker will mimic spontaneous cardiac activity and thus cause inappropriate inhibition of a demand pacemaker. Short periods of EMG inhibition are common and usually asymptomatic. Longer periods may cause syncope (*Figs.* 16.12, 16.13). By reducing pacemaker sensitivity or altering the mode to fixed rate or triggered the problem can be solved.

6. *Pacemaker mediated tachycardia*. Prolongation of the atrial refractory period of a 'universal' pacemaker will terminate this arrhythmia.

## PACING ELECTRODES

### Endocardial versus Epicardial Pacing

There are two methods of attaching a pacing lead to the heart. First, an electrode can be passed pervenously and attached to the endocardium. Secondly, during thoracotomy an electrode can be sutured to the epicardium.

The epicardial approach is now much the less popular because of the risks associated with thoracotomy and general anaesthesia and doubt about the long term reliability of epicardial pacing leads.

Electrode displacement, once a common problem, was the main reason for favouring epicardial pacing but, with improvement in electrode design, it is now rare.

### Endocardial Lead Fixation Devices

Over the past few years a number of different modifications to the transvenous lead tip have been made in order to prevent lead dislocation. These include the use of small fins, tines or a helix which are intended to become entrapped in the trabeculae of the right ventricle or right atrial appendage. Another fixation method is the coating of the electrode tip with a porous surface so that fibrous tissue quickly grows into the pores, affording fixation.

### Unipolar versus Bipolar Pacing

Bipolar leads have both cathode and anode at the tip of the lead whereas with a unipolar lead the anode is remote from the cathode, being incorporated into the pacemaker generator surface.

Unipolar lead systems are more widely used than bipolar systems. The small distance between electrodes in the bipolar system may result in failure to sense spontaneous cardiac activity, when of low amplitude, and consequent failure of demand pacing. The large distance between cathode and anode in unipolar lead systems facilitates much greater sensitivity, though one disadvantage is that extracardiac electrical signals, for example from skeletal muscle, may also be sensed and be misinterpreted as spontaneous cardiac activity, resulting in inappropriate inhibition of the pacemaker.

## IMPLANTATION OF A TRANSVENOUS SYSTEM

### Method

Implantation of a transvenous pacing system takes about 30 min and is usually performed under local anaesthesia. The pacing lead is introduced into the venous system by one of several routes: the most common are the cephalic vein, by direct cutdown, or subclavian vein puncture.

In the case of ventricular pacing, the lead is advanced to the apex of the right ventricle as described in Chapter 15. In the case of atrial pacing or sensing, the lead is introduced into the right atrial appendage. When a satisfactory position has been found the lead is attached to the pulse generator which is usually implanted subcutaneously over pectoralis major.

## Measurements

In order to ensure satisfactory pacing, at least two measurements must be made: the pacing threshold and the amplitude of the atrial or ventricular electrogram, whichever is to be sensed by the pacemaker.

The pacing threshold is the minimum strength of stimulation required to excite the heart consistently. It should be less than 1 V and 1 mA. The threshold increases after pacemaker implantation, often trebling within the few weeks after surgery. If the initial threshold is high, it is likely that the electrode tip is not in good contact with the endocardium and that the threshold may rise beyond the output of the pacemaker — usually about 5 V — causing exit block.

The threshold is affected by characteristics in both the pulse generator and lead. The duration of the pacing stimulus varies between pacemaker models. A short impulse duration involves the delivery of less energy to the heart and will therefore conserve battery life. On the other hand, the shorter the impulse duration, the higher the measured threshold will be. It is important to measure the threshold using stimuli of the same pulse duration as that of the pulse generator to be used. The most commonly used pulse duration is 0·5 ms.

The other measurement that must be made is the amplitude of the electrogram generated by the cardiac chamber from which sensing is carried out. In ventricular pacemakers the spontaneous intracardiac electrogram should be at least 3 mV. In atrial systems, which are more sensitive than ventricular systems, the atrial electrogram should be greater than 1·0 mV.

## Complications

Complications, which should be rare, are related either to the pacing lead or to the pulse generator.

Lead-related complications, such as dislocation, exit block, diaphragmatic stimulation and failure to sense, have been discussed in Chapter 15. They usually necessitate lead repositioning.

The main complications related to the generator are haematoma, infection and stimulation of the pectoral muscle beneath the pacemaker. It is unusual for antibiotic therapy to achieve long term cure of a pacemaker infection.

## FOLLOW-UP

Patients with pacemakers are seen at regular intervals for two main reasons. First, to ensure that the pacing system is working satisfactorily; secondly, to detect impending battery failure so that the pacemaker generator can be replaced before pacing stops. The most important signs of impending battery failure are a reduction in stimulation rate and an increase in impulse duration. Lithium-powered batteries give earlier warning of battery failure than did the older mercury—zinc cells.

### Electromagnetic Interference

Electromagnetic interference may mimic spontaneous cardiac activity and inhibit a demand pacemaker. In theory, a wide variety of domestic electrical apparatus can cause inhibition but in practice problems are minimal. At worst, interference is likely to cause the pacemaker to temporarily function in the fixed rate mode or to drop a couple of beats. In practice, patients should be told to avoid the immediate vicinity of old or poorly serviced microwave ovens and not to bend over running petrol or diesel engines. If by any chance they do experience palpitation or dizziness near to electrical apparatus they should promptly move a short distance away.

Anti-theft devices in shops and libraries can be triggered by pacemakers but are unlikely to cause the patient any problems. Patients should be advised not to dawdle at exit gates where these devices are in operation. Similar advice applies to weapon detector devices at airports, but pacemaker patients are usually allowed to bypass these systems.

Proximity to high powered radar installations and arc welding is contraindicated.

In patients who are likely to be exposed to strong electromagnetic fields during their employment, it is best to implant a pacemaker that can function in a triggered mode so that interference will cause modest acceleration rather than inhibition of the pacemaker. Where there is doubt about safety, ECG monitoring should be carried out at the place of work.

### Medical Equipment

Defibrillation may damage a pacemaker. Damage should be prevented by ensuring that the paddles are kept at least 15 cm from the pulse generator, though pacemaker function should be checked after defibrillation.

Diathermy may inhibit a demand pacemaker. Provided the equipment is kept as far away as possible from the pulse generator and the heart rhythm is monitored there should be no problems. Transurethral resection is often carried out in patients with pacemakers and, provided the above precautions are taken, there are no complications.

Short-wave heat treatment should not be applied to pacemaker patients.

### Driving Licences

In the United Kingdom patients with pacemakers are allowed to hold an ordinary driving licence provided that the pacemaker has been functioning satisfactorily for at least 3 months, that the patient regularly attends a pacemaker clinic and that the licensing centre has been notified. Patients with pacemakers are not allowed to hold a heavy goods vehicle or public service vehicle licence.

## Cremation

To avoid explosion, pacemakers must be removed before cremation.

## Main Points

1. Long-term pacing is indicated in almost all cases of symptomatic bradycardia and should also be considered in asymptomatic patients if there are high degrees of AV block or long pauses in sinus node activity.

2. Ventricular demand pacing prevents normal AV synchrony and does not permit a chronotropic response to exercise.

3. Loss of AV synchrony may cause symptomatic hypotension at rest (pacemaker syndrome) and can be prevented by atrial or AV sequential pacing.

4. Absence of a chronotropic response to exercise can markedly reduce exercise tolerance. Atrial synchronized ventricular pacing and rate responsive systems sensitive to physiological variables such as blood temperature, respiration or QT interval will facilitate a chronotropic response to exertion.

5. The modern pacemaker is small, reliable and has a long battery life. Pacemaker infection is the commonest reason for re-operation. Many other complications can be dealt with without reoperation if the pacemaker is programmable.

# Chapter 17

# Digoxin Toxicity

Digoxin toxicity is a common problem. Over 10 per cent of patients receiving the drug who are admitted to hospital have been found to have evidence of digoxin toxicity.

Several factors predispose to digoxin toxicity. These include impaired renal function, hypokalaemia, dehydration (often due to diuretics), age — the elderly are more susceptible to toxicity — and hypothyroidism. Quinidine, amiodarone and verapamil all increase digoxin levels.

A number of symptoms suggest digoxin toxicity. These include anorexia, nausea, vomiting, diarrhoea, mental confusion, xanthopsia and visual blurring. However, none of these symptoms is specific to digoxin toxicity; in patients with severe congestive heart failure in particular, gastrointestinal symptoms are often caused by heart failure rather than digoxin.

Digoxin toxicity can cause a number of disorders of cardiac rhythm. These include atrial tachycardia with AV block (*Fig.* 17.1), junctional

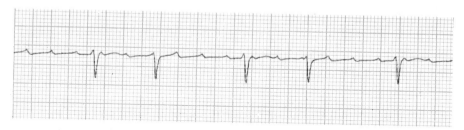

*Fig.* 17.1. Atrial tachycardia with varying degrees of AV block.

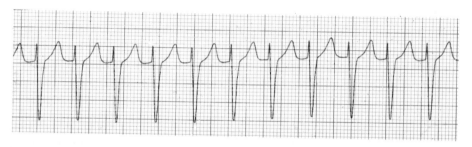

*Fig.* 17.2. Junctional tachycardia.

tachycardia (*Fig.* 17.2), ventricular ectopic beats (often bigeminy) (*Fig.* 17.3), ventricular tachycardia, first, second and third degree AV block, a slow ventricular response to atrial fibrillation (*Fig.* 17.4) and sino-atrial block (*Fig.* 17.5).

The main use of digoxin is to control the ventricular rate during atrial fibrillation. When a patient receiving digoxin for this purpose develops a regular pulse a number of possibilities should be considered. First, sinus rhythm may have returned. Secondly, an arrhythmia due to digoxin toxicity may have developed, e.g. atrial tachycardia with AV block, junctional tachycardia or atrial fibrillation with complete AV block. Without an ECG it may be difficult to ascertain whether the regular rhythm is due to an arrhythmia or not.

Plasma digoxin levels can be measured but must be interpreted in conjunction with clinical features. Levels less than 1·5 ng/ml, in the absence of hypokalaemia, indicate that digoxin toxicity is unlikely. Levels in excess of 3·0 ng/ml indicate that toxicity is probable. With levels between 1·5 and 3·0 ng/ml digoxin toxicity should be considered a possibility, particularly if there are symptoms or arrhythmias attributable to digoxin toxicity or if there is renal impairment, or if the patient appears to be on an inappropriately large dose of digoxin. Blood for digoxin concentration estimation must be taken at least 6 hours after the last dose.

## TREATMENT

Usually temporary discontinuation of the drug and correction of hypo-kalaemia, if present, are all that is required. Serious ventricular arrhythmias should be treated with intravenous anti-arrhythmic drugs. Lignocaine is suitable, though animal studies suggest that Epanutin (phenytoin) may be preferable. It has also been suggested that beta-blockers are particularly effective; these, however, may worsen AV node function and increase the risk of AV block developing.

If high degrees of AV block occur, temporary cardiac pacing may be necessary. Cardioversion is dangerous in the presence of digoxin toxicity. If cardioversion is essential, low energy levels, e.g. 5–10 Ws, increasing gradually as necessary, should be used and lignocaine 75–100 mg should be given.

In cases of acute overdosage gastric lavage should be carried out. A temporary transvenous pacemaker should be inserted since there is a high likelihood of AV block developing. The heart rhythm should be monitored and arrhythmias treated accordingly.

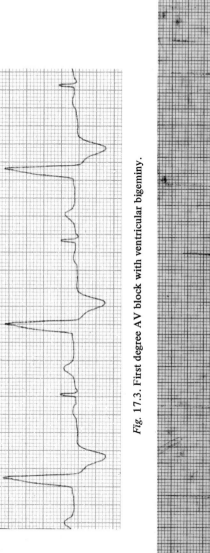

*Fig.* 17.3. First degree AV block with ventricular bigeminy.

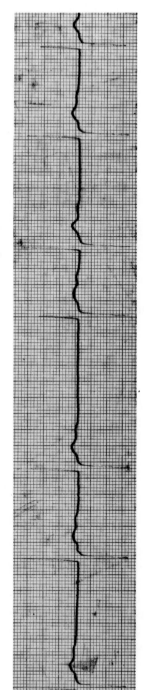

*Fig.* 17.4. Slow ventricular response to atrial fibrillation.

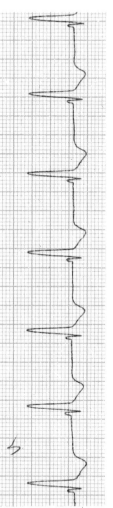

*Fig.* 17.5. Junctional escape rhythm resulting from sinus arrest.

## Main Points

1. Digoxin toxicity is common. Predisposing factors include impaired renal function, hypokalaemia, dehydration and some anti-arrhythmic drugs.

2. The most common symptoms are nausea and vomiting.

3. The most common arrhythmias are ventricular extrasystoles, atrial and junctional tachycardias and AV block.

4. Cardioversion is dangerous if there is digoxin toxicity. If essential, low energy shocks should be used.

5. Usually, temporary discontinuation of the drug is all that is required with re-introduction at a lower dosage after several days if digoxin is still required as in persistent atrial fibrillation.

# Chapter 18

# Ambulatory ECG Monitoring

Ambulatory ECG monitoring is now established as an invaluable diagnostic tool. The technique consists of continuously recording the ECG, usually for a period of 24 hours, on magnetic tape using a portable battery-operated tape recorder which is worn on a belt at the waist. If appropriate, the patient can be fully ambulant, carrying out his normal day-to-day activities.

The electrocardiogram is recorded by means of two electrodes applied to areas of thoroughly cleaned skin. Usually one electrode is placed over the manubrium sterni and the other electrode over the V5 chest lead position. As an alternative a modified V1 lead can be obtained by placing one electrode over the V1 chest lead position and the other electrode beneath the lateral part of the left clavicle. Some systems allow simultaneous recording of two leads. This increases diagnostic accuracy and aids in the detection of artefact which is unlikely to appear on both leads at the same time. Furthermore, sometimes one lead will not reveal important diagnostic information while another will (*see Figs.* 2.4, 6.22).

The tape recording is analysed in less than an hour by replaying it at 60–100 times real-time. Playback systems have facilities for printing out selected portions of the recording on ECG paper at standard speed. Most recording systems can automatically detect bradycardias, tachycardias and ectopic beats, though in practice it is necessary for an operator to supervise the analysis.

## CLINICAL APPLICATIONS

Only clinical applications will be discussed, though the technique is a valuable research tool. Ambulatory ECG monitoring has enabled the detection and diagnosis of intermittent disorders of cardiac rhythm thus elucidating the cause of symptoms such as syncope, palpitation and chest pain. The technique is most valuable when the patient actually experiences his usual symptoms during an ECG recording. The patient should be instructed to record the time of onset of his symptoms so that these can be correlated with the heart rhythm at that time. With some recorders the patient can operate an event marker which indicates the onset of symptoms on the tape. Even when the patient does not experience his symptoms during recording, rhythm abnormalities of diagnostic significance may be detected. Obviously, if the patient does not experience his symptoms during the recording and no rhythm abnormalities are found, an arrhythmic cause for the patient's symptoms cannot be excluded. It may be necessary to record several tapes before diagnostic information is obtained.

The technique has demonstrated that in patients with syncope but a normal routine ECG, sinus arrest is often, and complete AV block occasionally, the cause.

Ambulatory monitoring is of some value in assessing a patient's response to therapy. For example, not uncommonly a tape recording will reveal frequent ventricular arrhythmias in spite of the use of an anti-arrhythmic agent. One problem in using ambulatory monitoring to assess therapy is that there is a marked spontaneous variation in the frequency of arrhythmias and so on the basis of one tape, absence or improvement in arrhythmia may not necessarily be a consequence of drug therapy.

### 'NORMAL' FINDINGS

Sinus bradycardia, short pauses due to sino-atrial block and AV Wenckebach block can occur in normal people during sleep and should not be regarded as evidence of conduction tissue disease. These phenomena may also sometimes occur during the day in young people with high vagal tone.

Whereas a routine 12-lead electrocardiogram records approximately 60 heart beats, a normal 24-hour tape recording is likely to contain at least 90 000 beats. Thus, ambulatory electrocardiography is a very much more sensitive tool than a standard recording. For example, the finding of a single ventricular ectopic beat on a routine ECG suggests a much higher frequency than a hundred ectopic beats on a 24-hour tape. In fact, studies of apparently normal people using ambulatory electrocardiography have shown that unifocal ventricular extrasystoles occur quite commonly, as do supraventricular ectopic beats. Some studies have also found very short runs of relatively slow ventricular tachycardia in apparently normal young subjects.

### ARTEFACTS

A number of technical problems during ambulatory electrocardiography can result in what appear to be arrhythmias to the unwary.

If the tape speed slows for any reason, complexes will appear closer together and mimic tachycardia. However, the duration of each ventricular complex will be shorter than normal and this should alert the observer to the likelihood of artefact. Conversely, if the tape runs too fast, apparent bradycardia with broader than normal complexes will result.

Not infrequently, a lead will become disconnected during a recording: since no activity is being recorded the ECG will appear as a straight line and mimic sinus arrest. Furthermore, sometimes an electrical connection can intermittently fail, resulting in repeated episodes of apparent sinus arrest. However, if a lead becomes disconnected it is likely to do so at any point in the cardiac cycle, and it is unlikely that the onset of 'asystole' will arise after the ventricular T wave as it would if sinus arrest were real. If the onset of sinus arrest does occur during the inscription of an atrial or ventricular complex, artefact can be assumed.

Occasionally, artefact can produce an apparent tachycardia but close inspection will reveal that normal QRS complexes are 'walking through' the tachycardia.

## INFREQUENT PALPITATION

Patients with infrequent palpitation are unlikely to experience an episode during a 24-hour recording. Recently, a very useful and relatively inexpensive device (cardio-memo recorder) has been introduced which will record 30 s of electrocardiogram. The patient can carry the device around until an attack occurs. He or she then applies the device to the chest wall and activates the recording which is stored in a memory and can be replayed directly or via the telephone into an ECG machine.

Clearly, the device is not suitable for the investigation of episodes which disable the patient to the extent that they cannot activate the recorder. It is very important that it is explained to the patient precisely when and how to use the recorder.

# Main Points

**1.** Ambulatory electrocardiography is very useful for the investigation of syncope, near-syncope, palpitation and other symptoms thought to be due to an arrhythmia when routine electrocardiography has not provided diagnostic information.

**2.** Artefact can produce apparent arrhythmias but can usually be recognized by careful inspection of the recording.

**3.** Studies in apparently normal subjects have demonstrated that certain rhythm disturbances detected by ambulatory electrocardiography are not of pathological significance.

**4.** For patients with infrequent, non-disabling palpitation, provision of a cardio-memo recorder is the best method of investigation.

**5.** Useful information will be provided from an ambulatory recording, if an arrhythmia is demonstrated or if a patient experiences his usual symptoms without a disturbance in rhythm. Clearly if there is no arrhythmia and no symptoms, then an episodic arrhythmia has not been excluded.

# Chapter 19

# Intracardiac Electrophysiological Testing

Information derived from intracardiac electrophysiological testing has led to an increased understanding of conduction defects and tachycardias.

In the assessment of the individual patient, the technique has a limited role. Its main uses are for investigating the feasibility of pacing techniques or surgery for control of tachyarrhythmias. In addition, it is occasionally of value in detecting abnormal function of the sinus node or AV junction in patients with suspected conduction tissue disease in whom repeated standard and ambulatory electrocardiography has been uninformative. Similarly, in patients with infrequent palpitation in whom ambulatory electrocardiography has not provided diagnostic information, the technique can be used to try to initiate a tachycardia.

Here, discussion will be limited to a brief account of the technique and some of its uses.

## TECHNIQUE

The sequence of cardiac chamber activation, during normal and abnormal rhythms, is studied by recording electrograms from various intracardiac sites using transvenous bipolar electrodes which are introduced via femoral and antecubital veins, under local anaesthesia.

Activity from the right atrium, left atrium, ventricles and bundle of His can be recorded by positioning electrodes in the right atrium, in the coronary sinus (which passes behind the left atrium), right ventricle and across the tricuspid valve, respectively. The intracardiac electrograms together with surface leads are recorded simultaneously on a multi-channel recorder, usually at a paper speed of 100 mm/s (*Fig.* 19.1).

### His Bundle Electrogram

Careful positioning of an electrode across the tricuspid valve enables His bundle activity to be recorded (*Fig.* 19.1). Activity from the low right atrium and interventricular septum is also recorded. The three waves are designated H, A and V, respectively. The A−H interval indicates the time taken for an atrial impulse to be conducted through the AV node and the

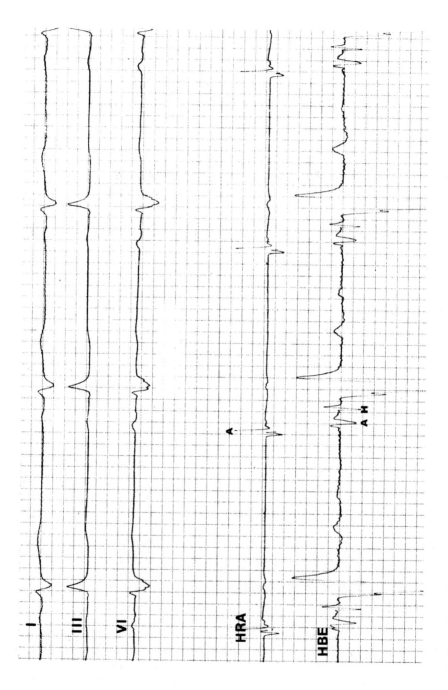

*Fig.* 19.1. Simultaneous recording, at 100 mm/s, of surface leads I, III and V1 together with a high right atrial electrogram (HRA) and His bundle electrogram (HBE). A, atrial activity; H, His bundle activity.

H–V interval represents the time taken for transmission through the bundle of His and the bundle branches to the ventricles.

## Pacing

The recording electrodes can also be used for atrial or ventricular stimulation. Two basic methods of pacing are employed: first, regular pacing at various rates; secondly, using a programmable stimulator, precisely timed premature stimuli can be introduced during spontaneous or paced rhythm (*see Fig.* 19.4). These can be timed to occur progressively earlier in the cardiac cycle so that the whole cycle is scanned. Sometimes double or triple stimuli are used.

## CLINICAL APPLICATIONS

### AV Conduction

In patients with complete heart block, knowledge of whether the block is at AV nodal or infranodal level may be of practical significance (*see* Chapter 9). In patients with AV nodal block the subsidiary pacemaker will be in the bundle of His and each ventricular complex will, therefore, be preceded by a His bundle spike (*Fig.* 19.2). On the other hand, when the block is infranodal, His bundle and ventricular activity will be dissociated.

The normal H–V interval, which is a measure of conduction time through the bundle of His and bundle branches, is 35–55 ms. Any increase indicates impaired conduction.

In patients with bifascicular block a prolonged H–V interval is evidence of slowed conduction in the functioning fascicle and means that there is trifascicular disease (however, prophylactic pacing of patients with trifascicular disease is not of proved benefit).

Occasionally, in patients with infrequent Stokes–Adams attacks, it may not be possible to establish the cause in spite of standard and continuous ambulatory electrocardiograms. Prolongation of the H–V interval strongly points to abnormal AV conduction, though a normal measurement does not exclude impaired conduction. Sometimes H–V prolongation can only be induced when the intraventricular conducting system is stressed by an atrial ectopic beat (*Fig.* 19.3).

### Sick Sinus Syndrome

Intracardiac electrophysiological testing may be useful in· patients in whom the sick sinus syndrome is suspected but cannot be proved by surface electrocardiography. In normal subjects cessation of rapid atrial pacing or single premature atrial stimuli leads to only a brief pause before sinus node activity resumes. In patients with sick sinus syndrome a profound depression of sinus node activity can result. When the 'sinus node recovery time' is greater than 140 per cent of the sinus cycle length,

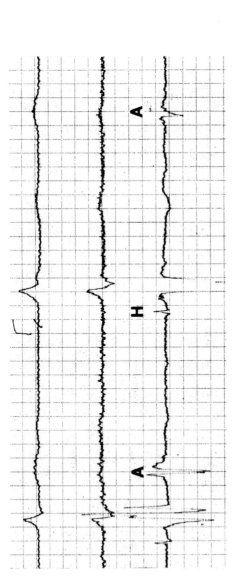

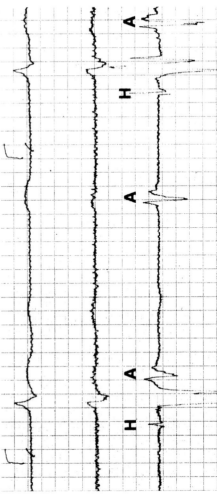

*Fig.* 19.2. Continuous trace: Complete heart block at AV nodal level. Simultaneous recording of two surface ECG leads and His bundle electrogram at 100 mm/s. Each ventricular complex is preceded by His bundle activity (H). Atrial activity (A) is dissociated from ventricular activity.

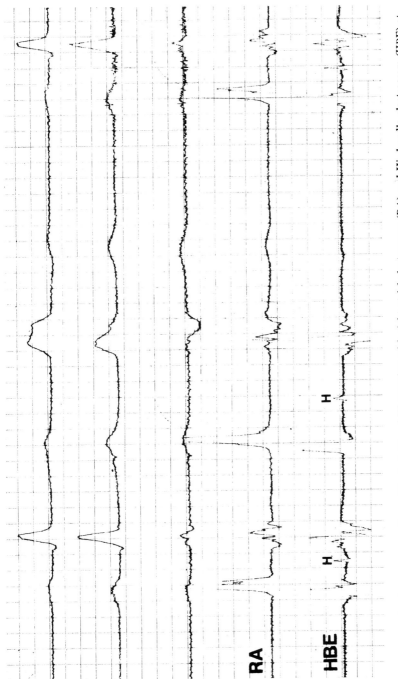

*Fig.* 19.3. Simultaneous recordings of leads I, II and III together with right atrial electrogram (RA) and His bundle electrogram (HBE) at 100 mm/s. The second complex is an atrial ectopic beat conducted with left bundle branch block. In this beat, the H–V interval is markedly increased at 140 ms.

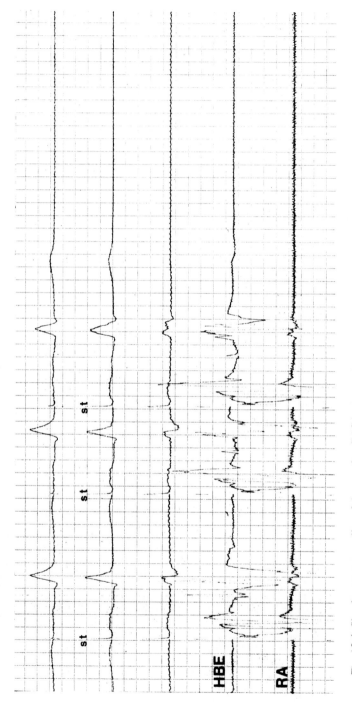

*Fig.* 19.4. Simultaneous recording of three surface ECG leads together with His bundle (HBE) and right atrial (RA) electrograms at 100 mm/s. Right atrial pacing stimuli (st) at regular intervals of 570 ms are followed by a single extrastimulus with a coupling interval of 340 ms. This resulted in total cardiac standstill over 5 s after which the pacemaker had to be re-started. The premature atrial stimulus also slightly increased the duration of the H−V interval.

sick sinus syndrome should be suspected. An extreme example is shown in *Fig.* 19.4.

An atrial pacemaker can only be used in cases of sick sinus syndrome if AV function is satisfactory. If second degree AV block develops at relatively low atrial pacing rates (e.g. less than 120/min) or if there is a prolonged H–V interval, atrial pacing is usually contraindicated.

## Atrial Activity During Tachycardia

A right atrial electrogram can sometimes be of great diagnostic help when atrial activity during tachycardia cannot be identified from the surface electrocardiogram (*Fig.* 19.5, 19.6).

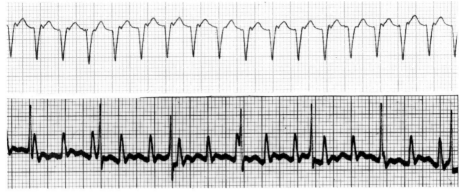

*Fig.* 19.5. Recording at 25 mm/s of lead V5 and right atrial electrogram in a patient with acute anterior myocardial infarction thought to have had paroxysmal supraventricular tachycardia. Atrial activity is slower than and dissociated from the ventricular activity indicating that the tachycardia is of His bundle or ventricular origin.

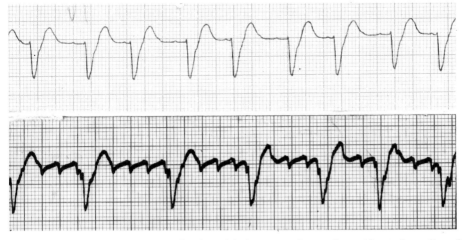

*Fig.* 19.6. Recording of lead V1 and right atrial electrogram in a patient with a tachycardia and left bundle branch block. The atrial electrogram shows atrial flutter, although this was not clear from any of the surface ECG leads.

## Paroxysmal Supraventricular Tachycardia

Paroxysmal supraventricular tachycardia can usually be initiated and terminated by precisely timed premature atrial or ventricular stimuli (*Fig.* 19.7, 19.8). The ability to stop and start tachycardias allows the effects of drugs and pacing techniques to be studied.

When surgery is being considered for paroxysmal supraventricular tachycardia it is important to know whether the re-entrant circuit is made up by a bundle of Kent or an additional intra-AV nodal pathway (*see* Chapter 6). Even in patients with the Wolff–Parkinson–White syndrome the tachycardia sometimes does not involve the bundle of Kent but is due to dual AV nodal pathways. Recording of the sequence of atrial activation during tachycardia usually enables distinction between the two mechanisms. In tachycardia due to dual AV nodal pathways, because the ventricular impulse re-enters the atria via the AV node, atrial activity will be first recorded by the His bundle electrode, since it is nearest to the AV node. On the other hand, if re-entry occurs via a left- or right-sided bundle of Kent, atrial activation will be recorded first in either coronary sinus or lateral right atrial electrograms. Many cases of paroxysmal supraventricular tachycardia without surface ECG evidence of pre-excitation have been shown to have a concealed left-sided bundle of Kent using this technique (*Fig.* 19.9).

## Atrial Fibrillation in the Wolff–Parkinson–White Syndrome

Atrial fibrillation in the Wolff–Parkinson–White syndrome can lead to a dangerously fast ventricular rate. The ventricular response to atrial fibrillation can be studied by inducing atrial fibrillation by rapid (250–1000 stimuli/min) right atrial pacing. If the ventricular rate is dangerously fast, the procedure can be repeated after administration of a drug to ensure that the ventricular response is slowed (*see* Chapter 7).

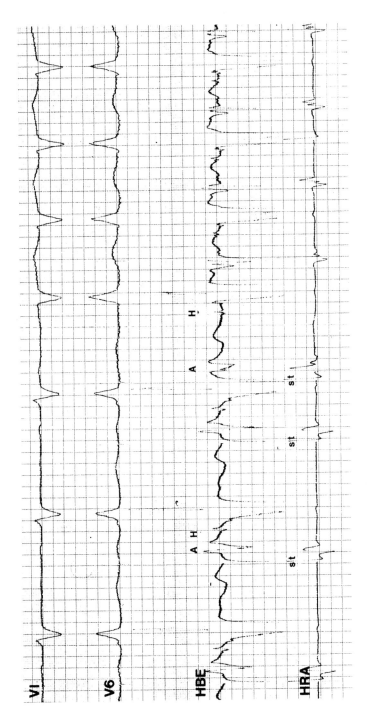

*Fig.* 19.7. Simultaneous recording of leads V1, V6, His bundle and high right atrial electrograms at 100 mm/s. The right atrium is being stimulated (st) at intervals of 530 ms after which an atrial extrastimulus with a coupling interval of 260 ms is introduced. The extrastimulus initiates supraventricular tachycardia.

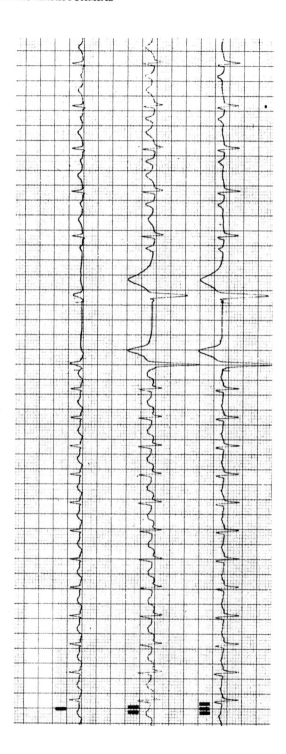

*Fig.* 19.8. Paroxysmal supraventricular tachycardia terminated by the first of two paced ventricular beats.

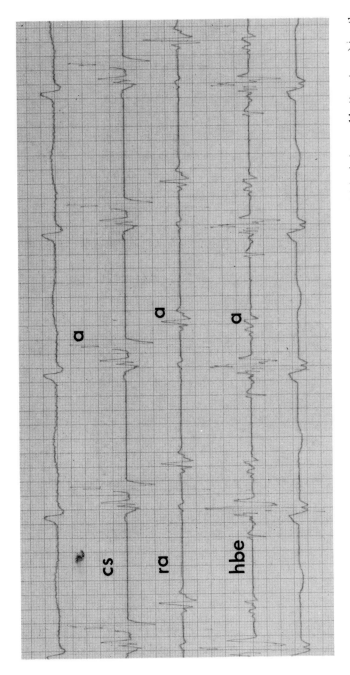

*Fig.* 19.9. Paroxysmal supraventricular tachycardia with simultaneous recordings of two surface ECG leads (top and bottom traces) together with coronary sinus (**cs**), right atrial (**ra**) and His bundle (**hbe**) electrograms. Atrial activity (**a**) in the coronary sinus electrogram (which reflects left atrial activity) precedes right atrial activity during the tachycardia, indicating that the re-entrant mechanism involves a left-sided bundle of Kent.

Chapter **20**

# Arrhythmias for Interpretation: a Quiz

In this chapter examples of a variety of arrhythmias are given. The 'answers' appear on pp. 189–193. As is often the case in practice, there may be more than one observation to make about each example.

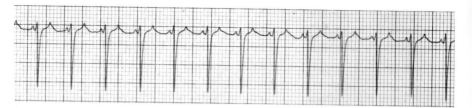

*Fig.* 20.1. Lead V1.

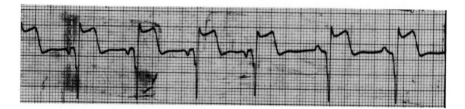

*Fig.* 20.2. Lead AVF.

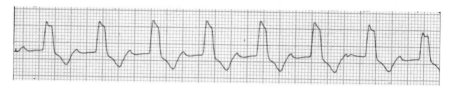

*Fig.* 20.3. Lead I.

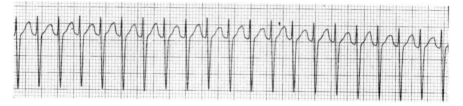

*Fig.* 20.4.

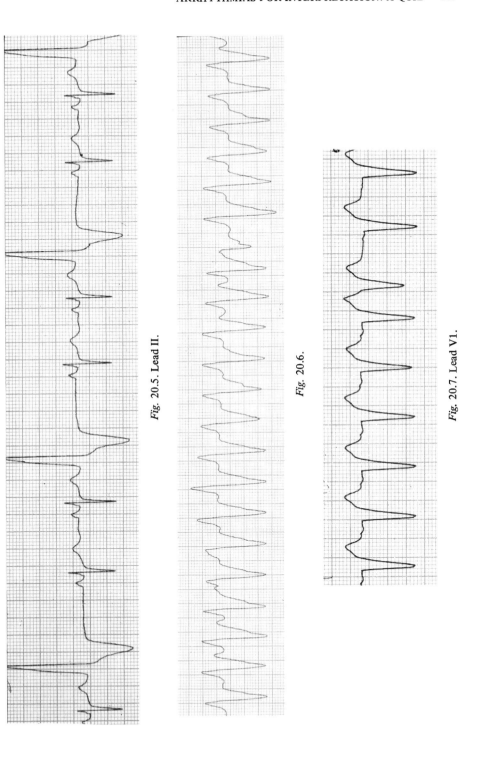

*Fig.* 20.5. Lead II.

*Fig.* 20.6.

*Fig.* 20.7. Lead V1.

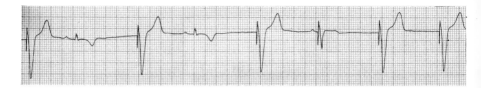

*Fig.* 20.8. Lead II.

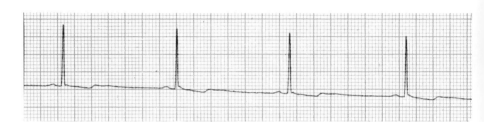

*Fig.* 20.9.

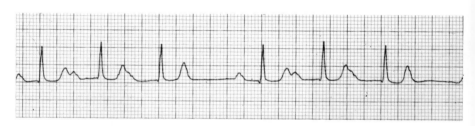

*Fig.* 20.10. Lead AVF.

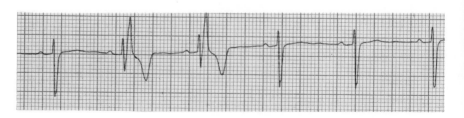

*Fig.* 20.11. Lead V1.

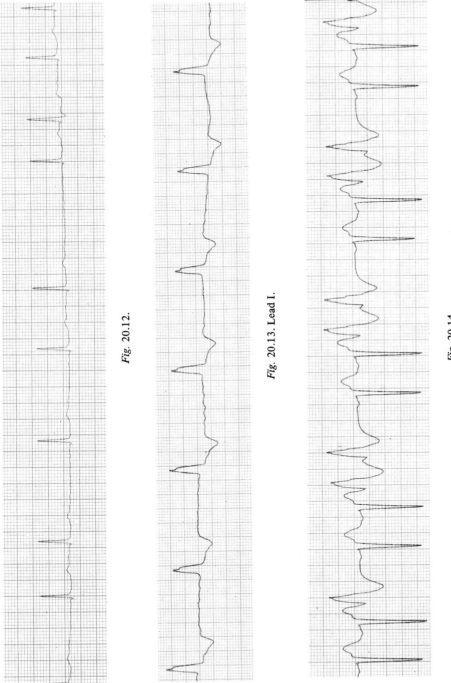

*Fig.* 20.12.

*Fig.* 20.13. Lead I.

*Fig.* 20.14.

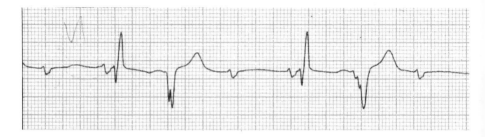

*Fig.* 20.15. Lead V1.

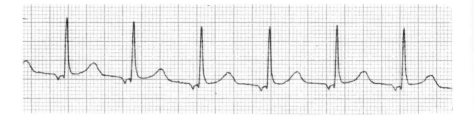

*Fig.* 20.16. Lead AVF.

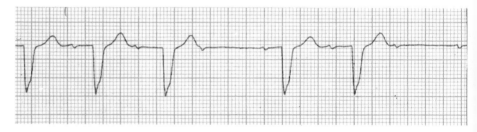

*Fig.* 20.17. Lead V1.

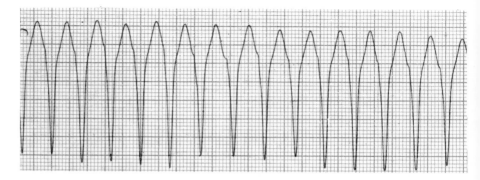

*Fig.* 20.18.

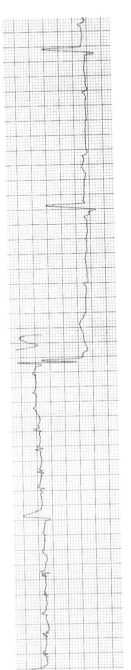

*Fig.* 20.19. Continuous recording as lead is changed from AVR to V1.

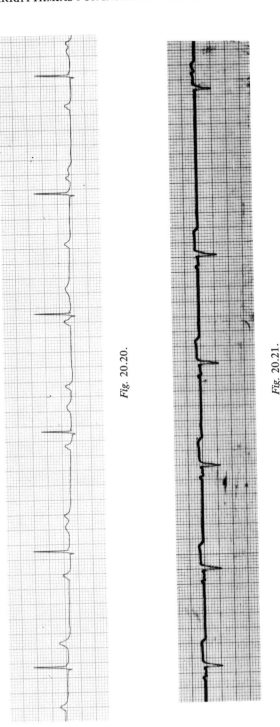

*Fig.* 20.20.

*Fig.* 20.21.

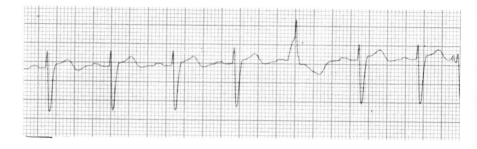

*Fig.* 20.22

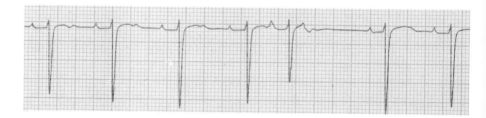

*Fig.* 20.23.

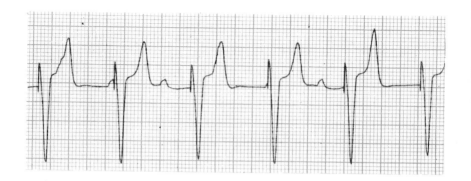

*Fig.* 20.24. Lead II.

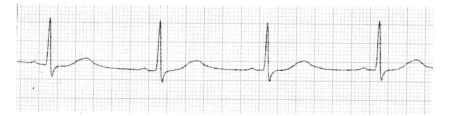

*Fig.* 20.25. Lead I.

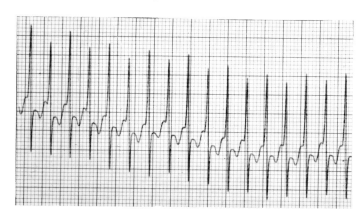

*Fig.* 20.26.

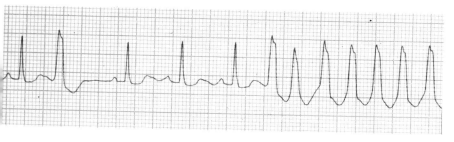

*Fig.* 20.27.

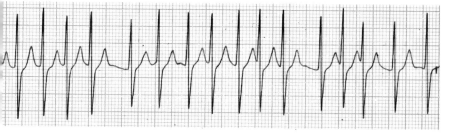

*Fig.* 20.28.

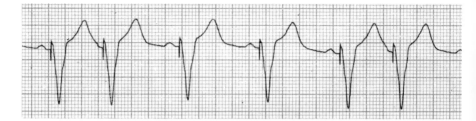

*Fig.* 20.29. Lead II.

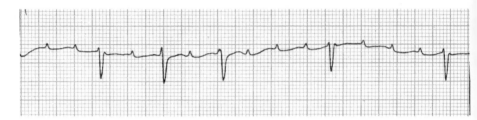

*Fig.* 20.30. Lead V1.

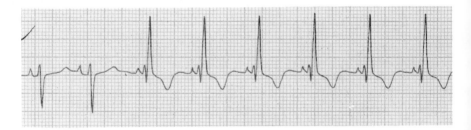

*Fig.* 20.31. Lead V1.

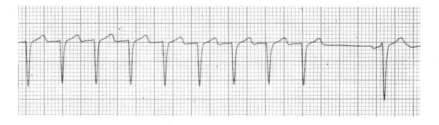

*Fig.* 20.32. Lead V1.

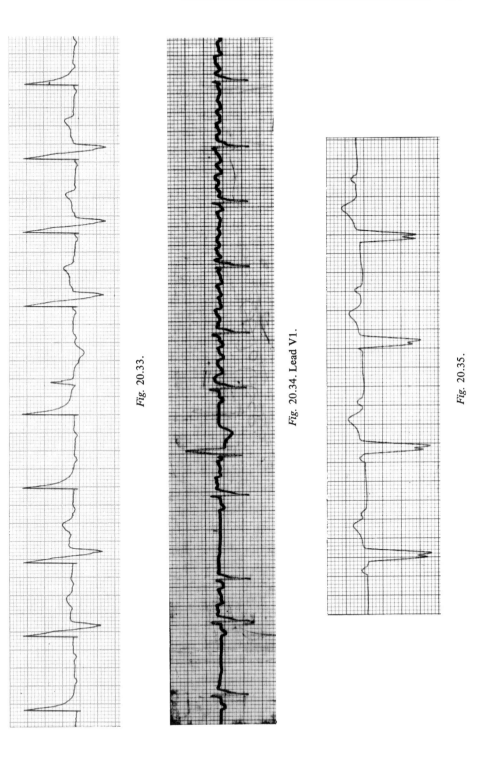

*Fig.* 20.33.

*Fig.* 20.34. Lead V1.

*Fig.* 20.35.

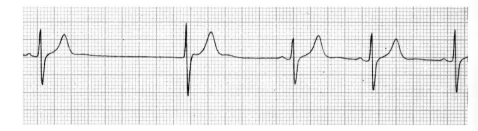

*Fig.* 20.36.

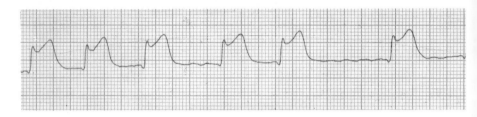

*Fig.* 20.37. Lead AVF.

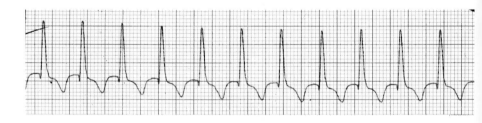

*Fig.* 20.38.

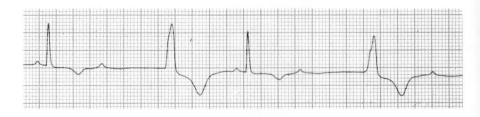

*Fig.* 20.39.

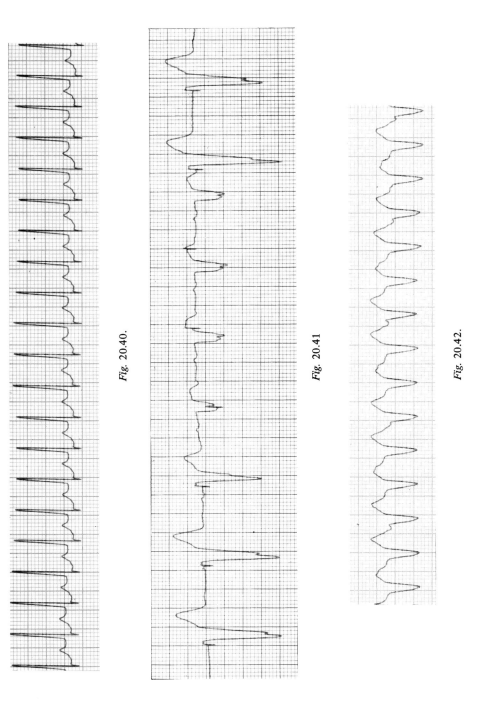

*Fig.* 20.40.

*Fig.* 20.41

*Fig.* 20.42.

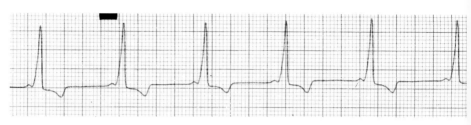

*Fig.* 20.43. Lead V6.

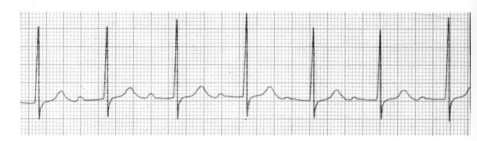

*Fig.* 20.44.

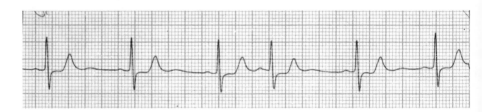

*Fig.* 20.45.

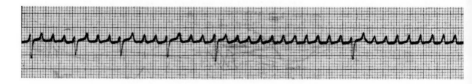

*Fig.* 20.46.

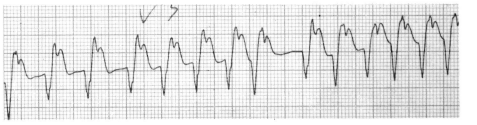

*Fig.* 20.47. Lead V3.

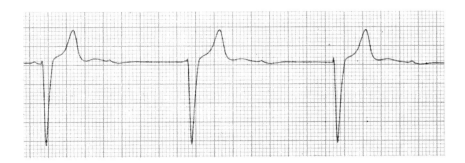

*Fig.* 20.48.

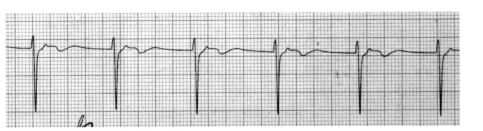

*Fig.* 20.49.

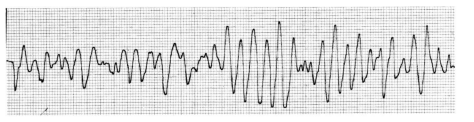

*Fig.* 20.50.

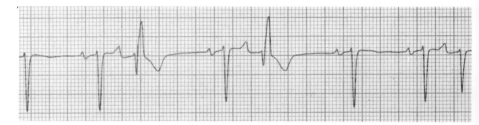

*Fig*. 20.51.   Lead V1.

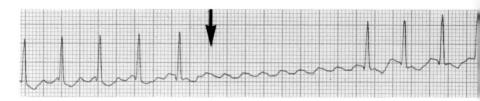

*Fig*. 20.52.   Arrow indicates carotid sinus massage.

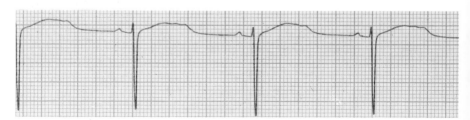

*Fig*. 20.53.

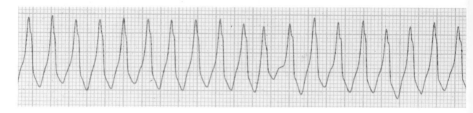

*Fig*. 20.54.

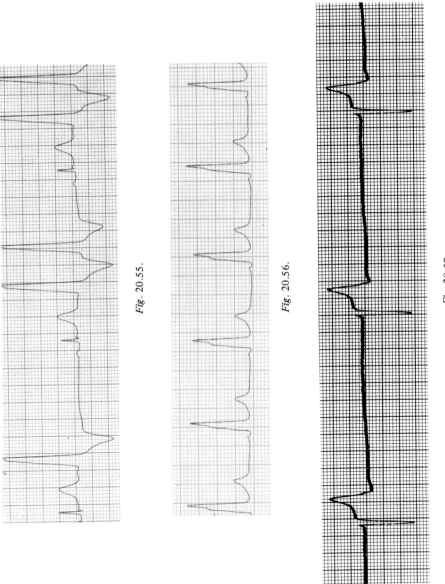

Fig. 20.55.

Fig. 20.56.

Fig. 20.57.

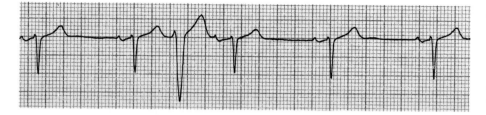

*Fig.* 20.58.

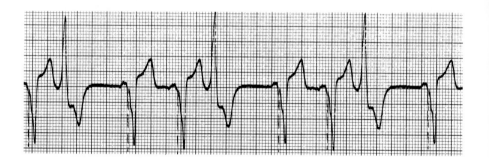

*Fig.* 20.59.

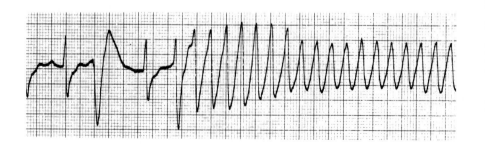

*Fig.* 20.60.

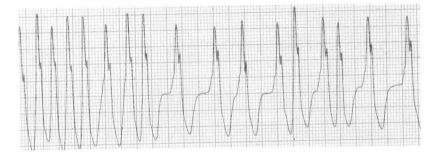

Fig. 20.61.

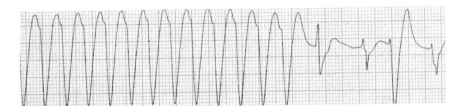

Fig. 20.62.

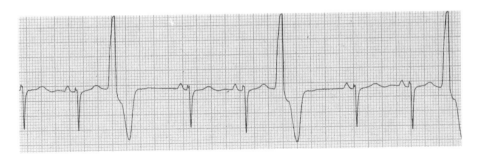

Fig. 20.63.

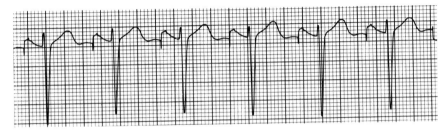

Fig. 20.64.

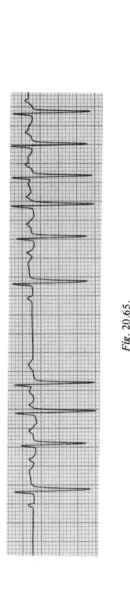

*Fig.* 20.65.

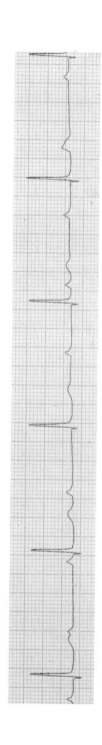

*Fig.* 20.66.

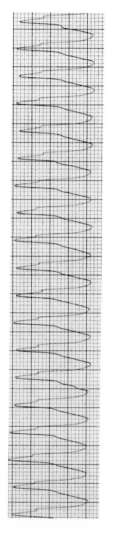

*Fig.* 20.67.

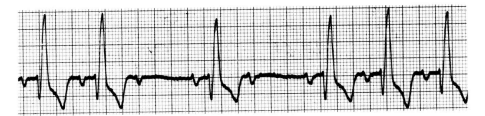

*Fig.* 20.68.

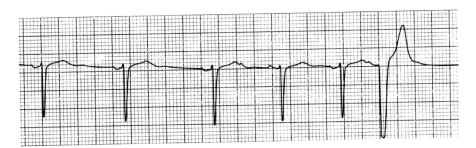

*Fig.* 20.69.

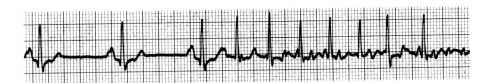

*Fig.* 20.70.

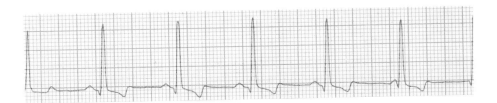

*Fig.* 20.71.

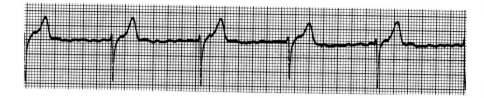

*Fig.* 20.72.

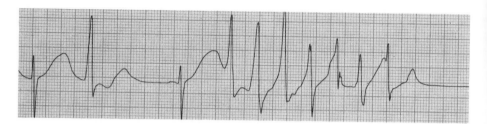

*Fig.* 20.73.

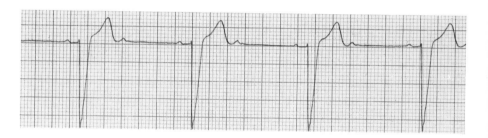

*Fig.* 20.74.

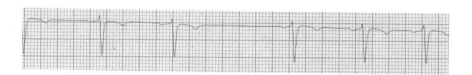

*Fig.* 20.75.

# ANSWERS

*Fig.* 20.1. Atrial flutter with 2 : 1 AV block.

*Fig.* 20.2. Inferior myocardial infarction. The first five beats are of junctional origin.

*Fig.* 20.3. Left bundle branch block with first degree AV block. A P wave is superimposed on the end of the preceding T wave.

*Fig.* 20.4. Paroxysmal supraventricular tachycardia.

*Fig.* 20.5. Sinus rhythm with ventricular trigeminy. The ventricular complexes during sinus rhythm are predominantly negative indicating left axis deviation.

*Fig.* 20.6. Ventricular tachycardia. The sixteenth beat is a fusion beat.

*Fig.* 20.7. Left bundle branch block as indicated by the broad QS complexes in lead VI. An atrial ectopic beat is superimposed on the T wave of the seventh beat and is also conducted with left bundle branch block.

*Fig.* 20.8. Ventricular demand pacemaker inhibited by sinus beats. The sixth complex is a fusion beat.

*Fig.* 20.9. Sinus bradycardia.

*Fig.* 20.10. AV Wenkebach phenomenon. The non-conducted beat is superimposed on the T wave of the preceding beat.

*Fig.* 20.11.  Intermittent right bundle branch block.

*Fig.* 20.12. Atrial fibrillation with slow ventricular response.

*Fig.* 20.13. Atrial fibrillation with complete AV block.

*Fig.* 20.14. Single and coupled ventricular extrasystoles.

*Fig.* 20.15. A 2 : 1 AV block with ventricular ectopic beats.

*Fig.* 20.16. Junctional rhythm. Each ventricular complex is preceded by an inverted P wave indicating that the junctional focus has also activated the atria.

*Fig.* 20.17. AV Wenkebach block with left bundle branch block.

*Fig.* 20.18. Ventricular tachycardia.

*Fig.* 20.19. V1 shows complete AV block. The apparent rapid atrial activity in lead AVR is caused by somatic tremor due to Parkinson's disease.

*Fig.* 20.20. Complete AV block with narrow ventricular complexes.

*Fig.* 20.21. Sinus bradycardia with sinus arrest followed by a junctional escape beat.

*Fig.* 20.22. Sinus rhythm with an end-diastolic ventricular ectopic beat.

*Fig.* 20.23. Atrial ectopic beat superimposed on fourth ventricular T wave.

*Fig.* 20.24. Ventricular pacing. Dissociated atrial activity can clearly be seen.

*Fig.* 20.25. Sinus bradycardia with prolonged QT interval (QTc = 0·53 s).

*Fig.* 20.26. Tachycardia of supraventricular origin with a rate of 290/min suggesting atrial flutter with 1 : 1 AV conduction.

*Fig.* 20.27. The second ventricular ectopic beat initiates ventricular tachycardia.

*Fig.* 20.28. Atrial fibrillation with rapid ventricular response.

*Fig.* 20.29. Atrial synchronous pacing. After the first and fifth ventricular complexes there are atrial extrasystoles which also trigger ventricular pacing.

*Fig.* 20.30. Atrial tachycardia with variable AV conduction.

*Fig.* 20.31. Sinus rhythm. Last six beats conducted with right bundle branch block.:.

*Fig.* 20.32. Paroxysmal supraventricular tachycardia which terminates after the ninth beat.

*Fig.* 20.33. Intermittent failure to capture of ventricular demand pacemaker: first, fourth, fifth and ninth pacing stimuli fail to capture ventricles. After fifth stimulus, spontaneous ventricular beat inhibits pacemaker indicating satisfactory sensing. In addition, there is an atrial tachycardia.

*Fig.* 20.34. Atrial ectopic beats follow the second, fourth and sixth ventricular complexes. The first ectopic beat is conducted normally, the second with right bundle branch block and the third leads to atrial fibrillation.

*Fig.* 20.35. Complete AV block with broad ventricular complexes.

*Fig.* 20.36. Following the first sinus beat there is sinus arrest and a junctional escape beat.

*Fig.* 20.37. Acute inferior myocardial infarction and atrial fibrillation with slow ventricular response.

*Fig.* 20.38. Junctional tachycardia.

*Fig.* 20.39. Second degree AV block with ventricular escape beats.

*Fig.* 20.40. Paroxysmal supraventricular tachycardia.

*Fig.* 20.41. Fixed rate ventricular pacing. The pacemaker is not inhibited by the period of sinus rhythm after the third paced beat.

*Fig.* 20.42. Ventricular tachycardia. There are peaks at regular intervals superimposed on the T waves of the first, fourth, seventh, tenth and thirteenth complexes which may be due to independent atrial activity.

*Fig.* 20.43.  Sinus rhythm with Wolff–Parkinson–White syndrome.

*Fig.* 20.44. First degree AV block. PR interval = 0·30 s.

*Fig.* 20.45. After the third sinus beat there is an atrial ectopic beat.

*Fig.* 20.46. Atrial flutter conducted with varying degrees of AV block.

*Fig.* 20.47. Atrial fibrillation in acute anterior myocardial infarction.

*Fig.* 20.48. Complete AV block. The third and fifth atrial impulses are concealed by ventricular complexes.

*Fig.* 20.49. Junctional rhythm with retrograde atrial conduction.

*Fig.* 20.50. Ventricular fibrillation.

*Fig.* 20.51.  Atrial ectopic beats superimposed on ventricular T waves of second, fourth and sixth ventricular complexes. The first two are conducted with right bundle branch block.

*Fig.* 20.52.  Atrial flutter with 2:1 AV block. Carotid massage causes transient complete AV block.

*Fig.* 20.53.  Sinus rhythm with long QT interval and prominent U waves (was due to amiodarone).

*Fig.* 20.54.  Ventricular tachycardia with capture beat.

*Fig*. 20.55.   Ventricular ectopic beats including couplets after second and third sinus beats.

*Fig*. 20.56.   Sinus rhythm with Wolff–Parkinson–White syndrome.

*Fig*. 20.57.   Sinus arrest. Ventricular escape rhythm.

*Fig*. 20.58.   Interpolated ventricular ectopic beat with retrograde concealed ventriculo-atrial conduction.

*Fig*. 20.59.   Atrial synchronized ventricular pacing. Two ventricular extrasystoles inhibit universal (DDD) pacemaker.

*Fig*. 20.60.   Second ventricular ectopic beat initiates ventricular flutter/fibrillation.

*Fig*. 20.61.   Atrial fibrillation. QRS morphology suggests delta waves, i.e. Wolff–Parkinson–White syndrome.

*Fig*. 20.62.   Paroxysmal ventricular tachycardia.

*Fig*. 20.63.   Ventricular trigeminy.

*Fig*. 20.64.   Atrial pacing.

*Fig*. 20.65.   Paroxysmal atrial tachycardia.

*Fig*. 20.66.   Complete AV block.

*Fig*. 20.67.   Ventricular tachycardia.

*Fig*. 20.68. Intermittent Mobitz II AV block.

*Fig*. 20.69.   Atrial ectopic beats superimposed on third and fifth ventricular T waves. First ectopic is not conducted, the second is conducted to the ventricles with left bundle branch block.

*Fig*. 20.70.   Paroxysmal atrial fibrillation.

*Fig*. 20.71.   AV dissociation.

*Fig*. 20.72.   Atrial fibrillation with complete AV block.

*Fig*. 20.73.   Sinus bradycardia with marked QT prolongation and short run of torsade de pointes tachycardia.

*Fig*. 20.74.   2:1 AV blocks. Conducted beats show left bundle branch block.

*Fig*. 20.75.   2:1 sino-atrial block.

# Index

aberrant intraventricular conduction 6, 45 (*figs.* 2.5–8, 6.5, 6.10, 6.15, 6.19)
ablation, transvenous 41 (*fig.* 6.8)
ambulatory ecg monitoring 154–6
amiodarone 111–12
antiarrhythmic drugs, clinical classification 106
antiarrhythmic drugs, action potential classification 106–7
artificial respiration 120
asystole 122
atrial ectopic beats (*see* ectopic beats)
atrial fibrillation 42–48, 61, 85, 97 (*figs.* 6.9–19, 11.11)
atrial fibrillation, causes 47
atrial flutter 48–52 (*figs.* 6.20–6.24)
atrial pacing 136 (*figs.* 15.4, 16.5)
atrial synchronized pacing 139–40 (*figs.* 16.9)
atrial tachycardia 52–55, 150 (*figs.* 6.25–6, 17.1)
AV block, second degree 73–5, 99, 133 (*figs.* 9.4–9.8 11.15)
AV block, in myocardial infarction 99–103
AV block, complete 75–6, 99–100, 132 (*figs.* 9.9–13, 11.16, 11.22)
AV block, first degree 72–3, 133 (*figs.* 9.1–9.3, 11.14)
AV dissociation 76 (*fig.* 9.14)
AV junction 7
AV re-entrant tachycardia 34–42, 59–61 (*figs.* 6.1–6.7, 7.7–9)
AV sequential pacing 139
axis deviation 21 (*fig.* 4.4)

beta-blockers 112
bifascicular block in myocardial infarction 100–3 (*figs.* 11.18–20, 11.22)
bifascicular block 79–80, 100–3 (*figs.* 9.15–17, 11.18–20)
bradycardia-tachycardia syndrome 85–6, 88 (*figs.* 10.5–7)
bundle branch block, left 19 (*figs.* 4.2, 9.17)
bundle branch block, right 18–19 (*figs.* 4.1, 11.18–20)
bundle of Kent 56

capture beats 26 (*figs.* 5.5, 8.5)
cardiac massage 120, 123
cardiac arrest 119–123
cardioversion 115–118, 27, 29
carotid sinus syndrome 89
carotid sinus massage 37, 68
compensatory pause 11 (*figs.* 2.3, 2.4)
concealed pre-excitation 61, 164 (*fig.* 19.19)
congenital heart block 81
coupling interval 4, 15

defibrillation 121–2
digoxin 113
digoxin induced arrhythmias 150–151 (*figs.* 17.1–5)
disopyramide 110
diving reflex 37–38

ectopic beats 4–14
ectopic beats, ventricular 8–14, 93 (*figs.* 2.4, 2.9–17, 11.4–7)
ectopic beats, atrial 6–7, 85, 95 (*figs.* 2.1, 2.5–8, 10.6)
ectopic beats, ventricular 8–14 (*figs.* 2.4, 2.9–17, 11.4–7)
ectopic beats, junctional 7–8 (*fig.* 2.2)
electromyographic inhibition 145 (*figs.* 16.12–13)
electromagnetic interference 148
embolism, systemic 47–8, 89
endotracheal intubation 120
escape beats and rhythms 15–17, 85 (*figs.* 3.1–2, 10.1–2, 10.4, 11.13)
exit block 130 (*fig.* 15.3)
extrasytoles (*see* ectopic beats)

fascicular block, posterior 23, 79 (*figs.* 4.7, 9.16)
fascicular block, anterior 21–23, 79 (*figs.* 4.5, 9.15)
flecainide 110
frontal QRS axis 21
fusion beats 27 (*figs.* 5.2, 5.6)

heart block, AV 72–82
heart block, congenital 81

heart block, sino-atrial 84 (*fig.* 10.3)
hemiblock 20–3
hexaxial reference system 20 (*fig.* 4.4)
His bundle electrocardiography
    157–9 (*fig.* 19.1)

idioventricular tachycardia 30, 95
    (*figs.* 5.9, 11.10)
implantable defibrillator 30
intracardiac electrophysiological testing
    135–45

Jervell and Lange-Nielsen syndrome 32
junctional tachycardia 54–5, 150
    (*figs.* 6.27, 17.2)

lignocaine 107–8
Lown–Ganong–Levine syndrome 63–4
    (*fig.* 7.11)

mexiletine 108
microshock 29–30
Mobitz I AV block 73–4 (*figs.* 9.4–5)
Mobitz II AV block 74–5 (*figs.* 9.6–9.7)

pacemaker generators 143
pacemaker syndrome 137 (*fig.* 16.7)
pacemaker, 'Universal' 140
pacing, demand 130, 134–136
    (*figs.* 16.3–4)
pacing, DDD 140, 143 (*figs.* 16.10–11)
pacing, AV sequential 130–1, 139
    (*figs.* 15.6, 16.8)
pacing, temporary 124–131
pacing, antitachycardia 39–41 (*fig.* 6.7)
pacing, 'rate responsive' 142
pacing, complications 129–130
    (*figs.* 15.3–5)
pacing, long-term 132–149
pacing, fixed rate 134–5 (*figs.* 16.1–2)
pacing, complications 129–130
parasytole 13 (*fig.* 2.17)
paroxysmal supraventricular tachycardia
    34–42, 59–61 (*figs.* 6.1–7, 7.7–9)
pre-excitation syndromes 56–64
premature contractions (*see* ectopic
    beats)
procainamide 109–10
programmable pacemaker 143–5

QT interval, hereditary prolongation
    32–33

QT interval 32–33 (*fig.* 5.11)
quinidine 109

Romano–Ward syndrome 32

sick sinus syndrome 83–89
sino-atrial disease (*see* sick sinus
    syndrome)
sinus arrest 83–4 (*figs.* 10.1–2)
sinus arrhythmia 3 (*fig.* 1.6)
sinus bradycardia 2, 83, 155, 98
    (*figs.* 1.4, 11.12)
sinus rhythm 1–2 (*figs.* 1.1, 1.2)
sinus tachycardia 2 (*fig.* 1.5)
sotalol 113
Stokes–Adams attacks 80–1
subclavian vein puncture 125–6
supernormal conduction 76 (*fig.* 9.13)
supraventricular tachycardia, paroxysmal
    34–42 (*figs.* 6.1–6.7)

tocainide 109
torsade de pointes tachycardia 30–32
    (*fig.* 5.10)

vagal stimulation 37–38
ventriculophasic sinus arrhythmia 75
ventricular tachycardia 24–33, 65–71, 95
    (*figs.* 5.1–5.8, 8.3–8.7, 8.9, 11.7–9)
ventricular fibrillation 90–95 (*figs.* 2.10,
    11.1–2)
ventricular ectopic beats (*see* ectopic
    beats)
ventricular tachycardia, atrial activity
    during 25, 67 (*figs.* 5.4–5.6, 8.4, 8.5)
ventricular flutter 92 (*fig.* 11.3)
ventricular tachycardia, torsade de
    pointes 30–32 (*fig.* 5.10)
ventricular tachycardia, causes 24
verapamil 39, 112

Wenkebach block (*see* AV block)
Wolff–Parkinson–White syndrome, AV
    re-entrant tachycardia 59–61
    (*figs.* 7.7–9)
Wolff–Parkinson–White syndrome 56–63
    (*figs.* 7.1–7.8)
Wolff–Parkinson–White syndrome, atrial
    fibrillation 58–59, 61–3, 164 (*figs.* 6.16,
    7.4–6)